Self-help for Mind and Body

Jane Bird and Christine Pinch

Newleaf

Newleaf

an imprint of
Gill & Macmillan Ltd
Hume Avenue
Park West
Dublin 12
with associated companies throughout the world
www.gillmacmillan.ie

© 2002 Jane Bird and Christine Pinch
0 7171 3422 9
Index compiled by Grainne Farren
Print origination by Carole Lynch, Dublin
Printed by ColourBooks Ltd, Dublin

*The paper used in this book is made from the wood pulp
of managed forests. For every tree felled, at least one tree
is planted, thereby renewing natural resources.*

A catalogue record is available for this book
from the British Library.

3 5 4 2

CONTENTS

Contents

Contents

DISCLAIMER

Whilst all the information in this book is given in good faith, neither the authors not the publisher is able to accept responsibility for the health of the reader or user. If you have any medical condition at all, please consult your medical adviser.

FOREWORD

A comprehensive technique for relaxation and personal transformation, Autogenic Therapy (also known as Training) consists of a series of simple mental exercises designed to turn off the body's 'fight or flight mechanism' and turn on restorative rhythms and harmonising associated with profound psycho-physical relaxation. Practised daily it can bring results comparable to those achieved by serious meditators. Yet unlike meditation, Autogenic Therapy has no cultural, religious or cosmological overtones. It demands no special clothing, unusual postures or practices. When you practise Autogenic exercises, emotional and spiritual renewal occurs in much the same way as physical renewal does when you detoxify the body. Its founder Dr Johannes Schultz discovered, as have those of us who have practised it since, that in a state of passive concentration all activity is governed by the autonomic nervous system, once believed to be out of man's control, and can be influenced by the person himself.

This happens not by exercising any *conscious* act of *will* but rather by learning to abandon oneself to an ongoing organismic process – entering into a state of *passive concentration*. This strange paradox is self-induced passivity and is central to the way Autogenic Therapy works its wonders. It is a skill which Eastern Yogis, famous for their ability to resist cold and heat, change the rate of their heartbeat, levitate, and perform other extraordinary feats of long practice use. But until the development of bio-feedback and Autogenic Therapy, and the arrival of Easter meditation techniques, this passive concentration largely remained a curiosity in the West, where active, logical, linear, verbal thinking, has been encouraged to the detriment of practising our innate ability to simply *be*. Many experts on the psychological processes of ageing believe it is this over-emphasis on the use of the conscious will in the western world that makes us highly prone to premature degeneration and stress-based illness in the first place.

Jane Bird and Christine Pinch have written an excellent book on Autogenic Therapy which fills a gap in the available literature about this important technique in English. A fascinating and thorough introduction to Autogenic Therapy for anyone considering learning it with a therapist, it is also an invaluable reference book for those who already practise the techniques. It is also a great resource for health professionals wanting to refer their patients to the professional therapy courses of the British Autogenic Society. I cannot praise the book highly enough and wish it God speed.

Leslie Kenton

ACKNOWLEDGMENTS

The authors would like to acknowledge, first, each other. Perhaps it is thanks to the very method of AT itself which has made it possible to complete this book with nothing but healthy disagreement and an ability to listen to and encourage each other. Our firm friendship remains intact, much to our relief!

We thank one of the Patrons of the British Autogenic Society, Leslie Kenton, for her valuable and much appreciated foreword. We would like to extend our thanks to the Chairperson Dr Janet Marshall and all members of the Executive Committee of the British Autogenic Society, which has endorsed this book. In addition, thanks to our many colleagues and friends from whom we have learned so much. In the therapy world, especially the 'autogenic world', it is often difficult to pinpoint the origin of an idea or concept, when working consistently with a creative and vibrant group of people. Many ideas have 'rubbed off' on us as we seek to improve our own autogenic practice with clients and the BAS therapist professional training.

We hold in special regard the Education and Training Team of the BAS, notably Dr Ann Bowden, Tamara Callea, Colin Marsh with all of whom we have worked closely for 10 years. We would add to these Dr Brian O'Donovan, Brian Davidson, and Dr Alice Greene – all past Chairpersons of the British Autogenic Society. Also thanks to Vera Diamond (under whose wise instruction Jane underwent Autogenic Neutralisation), and Tamara Callea for their help with Chapter Eleven.

Jane Bird thanks her sister Kate Ker (a highly experienced AT therapist and author) for introducing her to AT all those years ago – I never imagined it would lead to this! And she is eternally grateful to her friend and colleague Dr Roger Neighbour (now a Patron of the BAS in his capacity as sometime Chief Examiner for the Royal College of General Practitioners), who has been a strong support and fount of wisdom since 1983.

A big thank you to our families for their patience and tolerance over the years. To Jane's husband Martin and children Eleanor, William and Oliver, and to Chris's husband David and her children Daniel and Vicky, without whose unfailing interference this book might never have been finished!

We also thank all the hundreds of clients who have passed through our practices to learn AT. We are honoured and privileged to have witnessed their autogenic processes: without them we could not have learned our craft - and the learning goes on.

INTRODUCTION

Autogenic Therapy is an astonishingly simple form of self-help which can have very powerful effects. It is a method of easy mental exercises developed in Germany during the 1920s by the neurologist and psychiatrist, Dr Johannes Schultz. The exercises consist of the silent repetition of specific phrases, which, combined with the use of comfortable yet well-defined physical postures (sitting or lying), bring about a state of deep relaxation and mental calming. You learn to switch off the stressed 'fight, flight and freeze response' — changing from a state of alert activity to one of passive being.

Read any good book on complementary medicine, or stress, and you will see reference made to Autogenic Therapy as one of the best self-help therapies around. There may even be vague instruction on how to practise it. But there is a distinct shortage of authoritative writing, in English, by experienced autogenic therapists.

This book aims to fill the gap. It will tell you all about AT: the six standard exercises, explained in detail with their rationale, origins and development; the principles of self-regulation of the human organism; how emotions affect our health and what we can do about that. We will take you on a journey through a course, and explain both the therapist's role and that of the trainee.

In addition, we will present the history of AT, and provide an overview of some of the many research papers which, over the years, have been published in many countries. These demonstrate the efficacy of AT in a very wide area of application.

This is not, however, a 'teach-yourself-manual'. It would be folly to embark on learning AT without the guidance of a trained therapist, to monitor and support the process. At best, you might achieve a mere fraction of the potential benefit, missing out on the subtleties and detail of the autogenic process. At worst, you might cause yourself discomfort or distress.

THE AUTHORS

The authors of this book have, between them, over thirty years' experience of teaching AT.

Jane Bird *has worked with Autogenic Therapy in private practice, industry and the National Health Service, since 1983. Working as a trained nurse, and bringing up a family, she was looking for something 'to stop me sliding down a slippery slope'. She not only gained benefit for herself and her family (she stopped yelling at the kids; and has much better general health), but she also gained an enduring fascination with the innate, largely untapped powers of self-healing available in all of us. She followed up the basic eight-week course by undergoing Autogenic Neutralisation. Still working for the NHS, she was increasingly frustrated by the limitations of the nursing profession. She trained as an autogenic therapist in 1982, on a course largely led by Dr Wolfgang Luthe (Schultz's one-time colleague). Jane is a Founder Member of the British Autogenic Society.*

Chris Pinch *has taught AT for fifteen years in private practice, for industry and for a complementary health centre. She is a Registered General Nurse and has lectured in health education and human development. She learned AT following a turbulent period in her life. She felt, at 30-something, that she was getting old, assailed by aches and pains and lack of energy, and not realising that she was 'suffering from stress'. She feels that AT set her free from relying on others for her health and well-being, and she was intrigued by the possibilities of passing on to others the tools for self-help.*

Both Chris and Jane are tutors for the BAS and have been involved in developing therapist training programmes.

AUTOGENIC — THE MEANING

The word 'autogenic' means 'self-generating', or 'generated from within'. Derived from the Greek 'auto — self' and 'gen — produce', this can be interpreted in two ways. First, in practical terms, it can be taken to mean that the person learns the exercises and applies the therapy to themselves. Secondly, it can be interpreted as meaning that the results are spontaneous, derived from our inherent, self-regulating mechanisms — i.e. 'autogenic'. Significant positive outcomes can be achieved where AT has been taught and monitored by a knowledgeable and professional therapist.

AUTOGENIC THERAPY AS A STRESS MANAGEMENT TRAINING

How often have you heard it said: 'It's only stress — just go away and relax'? There is no doubt that relaxation should play a much larger part in our lives than it does. But the suggestion is often frustrating and unhelpful unless you know how to do it. AT is invaluable in helping a person to handle the normal stresses and strains of life. It is also used to treat physical and emotional symptoms that have their origins in stress, and for illnesses exacerbated by stress. AT is most certainly a skill for life.

AUTOGENIC THERAPY AS SELF-DEVELOPMENT

When we are in a state of good physical and emotional health, there is freedom to develop our potential for personal growth through enhanced creativity, physical fitness, mental ability, social contact, spirituality and aesthetic appreciation. Many people use AT to enhance these areas of their lives.

AUTOGENIC THERAPY AS THERAPY

Autogenic Therapy is often described as an effective form of psychotherapy. Certainly its deeper-level processes can bring profound understanding and insight. Basic AT can be a superb form of 'brief therapy'. It is not always necessary to 'get to the bottom' of a problem and understand its origin, in order for benefit to be gained. The concept of passive acceptance is sometimes enough for people to make changes quite spontaneously in their lives.

AT therapists experience real job satisfaction. The basic exercises are the same for everyone. The individual response is unique, and how that unfolds makes the process a truly fascinating one.

Above all, this book is about the human condition, and what we can do for ourselves to optimise our physical and psychological health and well-being.

> The goal of autogenic psychotherapy is that the patient acquires the necessary skill as far as possible uninfluenced by the therapist and is in this way able to form his own auto rhythm ... Schultz emphasised that trance effectuated [*sic*] with our method is **a safe way** to the altered state of consciousness.
>
> From Professor Heinrich Wallnöfer's Schultz Lecture,
> British Autogenic Society Seminar 2000

So — read on, and enjoy.

CHAPTER 1

WHAT IS AUTOGENIC THERAPY?

*A*utogenic Therapy is a simple method of self-healing, and, once learned, is a skill for life. Many people find that attending an AT course has been such a powerful experience that they have made permanent life changes even if they drop back in their practice in the years to come.

Autogenic Therapy (sometimes known as Autogenic Training) uses relaxation. The special mental exercises allow entry into an altered state of consciousness for a few minutes at a time. In Chapter 10 we will explain in more detail the background and development of the method. Suffice it to say here that Autogenic Therapy is now widely used in many parts of the world, and there are reputedly over 3,000 research papers which validate its efficacy in many different areas.

We all know that we should relax more. Relaxation is of great benefit to the human organism. The ability to let go, and move our conscious state into one of sleep, is a blissful experience. We seek this out every night, and we know the consequences if we don't. When we go on holiday, we may find that, after an adjustment period, we can lie in the sun doing nothing — without a care in the world. This is perhaps as near as many people get to a deep relaxation state, unless they use specific techniques.

The problem is that we do not generally allow ourselves time to relax. When the doctor or colleague tells us, 'Go away and relax', we probably associate this with taking an hour off, lying flat on the floor with a mask over our eyes, putting on a special CD with the sounds of birds, sea or wind in the trees, taking deep breaths and struggling to stay awake. Nice as this sounds, it takes up time we think we do not have, so we are put off before we even begin. Or we lie there reviewing our worries, getting even more agitated.

Many studies have been done which show how effective relaxation is, when it comes to our physical and emotional well-being. In the USA, the Mind/Body Medical Institute in Boston runs courses for chronic stress-related symptoms, including headache, fatigue and anxiety. The courses are from seven to thirteen weeks in duration, and use Benson's relaxation methods.

The results of this work, with 7,800 patients, showed approximately:

- 50 per cent reduction in general visits to the GP
- 36 per cent reduction in general visits to the GP by sufferers of chronic pain
- 80 per cent reduction in, or elimination of, medication for high blood pressure
- 75 per cent reduction in, or elimination of, medication for sleep disorders (Charlotte Broms: Workshop for British Autogenic Society, 1999)

Autogenic Therapy is often described as one of the following:

- Self-help for mind and body
- Easy mental exercises
- Profound relaxation
- A 'Western' meditation
- Good for you.

All of the above statements are essentially correct, and yet it is very difficult to describe succinctly exactly what Autogenic Therapy is, or what it has the potential to achieve.

Autogenic Therapy is a method which uses easy mental exercises to bring about a meditative state of mind and profound physical relaxation. You learn to apply these exercises to your everyday life. Practising them allows the mind/body system to switch itself out of the stress 'fight, flight and freeze' mode and into its opposite — 'relaxation, recuperation and restoration'.

Autogenic Therapy is a unique, non-invasive, non-drug approach to better health and well-being.

Using AT, you can achieve inner peace, and restore harmonious functioning in mind and body. You can boost your immune system, helping to prevent problems from colds to cancer. You can reduce risk factors in the cardiovascular system by reducing high blood pressure and cholesterol levels. You can use AT to heal yourself: post-operatively, emotionally and post-trauma. You can increase your self-confidence by becoming more self-aware and assertive. You can improve your sleep patterns and your relationships, reduce anxiety and cope with stress. You can improve your performance in work, the creative and performing arts, study and sport. Above all, you can take care of yourself very easily and enhance your quality of life, releasing your developmental potential.

A colleague of ours, Dr Riva Ripstein-Soicher, from Montreal, Canada, first heard of AT in 1977, when a brochure was sent to all General Practitioners in the province of Quebec, offering a training course in Autogenic Therapy by Dr Wolfgang Luthe (see Chapter 10). Her first reaction on reading it was to wave it over the bin, thinking, 'This sounds too good to be true. My mother always said, "Do not trust anything which is too good to be true."' However, Riva's curiosity won through as she reflected on how many of her patients suffered chronic symptoms from stress. She attended the course.

Riva's first attempt at teaching AT, to a hostile and disbelieving insomniac, brought about a surprising phone call after only four days of using the exercises: '*Madame — je dors* (I sleep).' Dr Ripstein-Soicher has been teaching AT in her practice ever since.

Although Autogenic Therapy is often proposed as a relaxation therapy, it is, in fact, much more than that. Any deep relaxation or meditative technique will initiate a release of physical and emotional sensations. These are related to the discharge of residual emotional material or physical tension or trauma which has been repressed. If you have ever felt tearful following a deeply relaxing treatment, or developed a cold as soon as you get on holiday, you have experienced something similar.

Autogenic Therapy allows and encourages this therapeutic release, enabling a swift process of readjustment that can bring about improvement of many symptoms in weeks or months. Using other psychological approaches, this work may take years.

The word 'autogenic' means 'self-generating'. It is derived from the Greek: 'auto — *self* and 'gen — *produce*'. There are two ways in which 'autogenic' can be interpreted:

1 *The exercises are self-administered.* Although you need a therapist to teach you the method, you actually carry out the treatment yourself. There is nothing 'hands-on' — no pills or scalpels.
2 *The autogenic response is self-generated.* Its therapeutic effects are generated from within, tapping into a person's unique self-healing system.

Once mastered, AT is always available without the need for a therapist or any equipment.

PREVENTION OF ILLNESS

The World Health Organisation describes good health as an optimum state of being which includes physical, emotional, mental, spiritual, social and sociological health.

People are now realising the importance of taking responsibility for their own health and well-being. We know that good diet, exercise and a healthy lifestyle can do a lot to prevent illness. Yet all too often we do nothing about our health until things go wrong; then we call upon our over-stretched health services, expecting treatment to get rid of our symptoms. Waiting times for treatment can often lead to deterioration of general health and well-being.

Drug therapy can, at times, be invaluable, but it can be overused, sometimes as a substitute for more time-consuming and expensive therapy. We know that the effectiveness of antibiotics is diminished with overuse, and side effects of medication can be unpleasant.

Autogenic Therapy can be used to support and enhance progress in other therapies. It has been clinically applied over a wide range of disorders.

SELF-RIGHTING MECHANISMS

Our greatest health resource is an intricate and complex system, which is innate in every human organism. We have an amazing capacity to recover from illness and injury. Look at how a simple cut finger can heal itself. When we break a bone in our leg, it is stabilised in plaster. Usually no other intervention is necessary in order to heal the bone. Similarly, think how ill we feel when we have the flu. But we recover — back to normal after a few days.

When things are going well and we are reasonably stress-free, there is a constant re-balancing going on within us. Our immune systems attack potentially harmful organisms; our blood pressures and pulses rise with exertion and return to normal all on their own.

These examples focus on the body, our physical being. We should not neglect the mind when discussing healing. If left to its own devices, the body will heal itself — so will the mind.

For example, we all know how much better we feel after a 'good cry'; an argument may clear the air; it's good to talk a problem through.

When we are overwhelmed by stress (di-stress) we rarely give ourselves the time needed to recuperate — the self-righting mechanisms can't keep pace, and eventually are unable to respond appropriately. Then symptoms begin. A vicious circle emerges, usually based on treatment of symptoms with no acknowledgement of underlying causes.

Learning AT can short-cut the time needed for recuperation by allowing you to switch regularly into 'recovery mode' for a few minutes at a time. *It may not be possible to change the things going on* around you, but you can learn how to change your reaction/response to stressful situations.

SUMMARY

Autogenic Therapy is an extremely effective self-help mind and body therapy which can influence many areas of health — giving greater control over physical health; improving emotional well-being; enhancing personal relationships; releasing creativity; providing coping skills; facilitating spiritual growth; and helping to fulfil true potential.

AUTOGENIC THERAPY — STANDARD EXERCISES

In his creation and development of AT, Schultz found a method which did not depend on a specialised symptom-based approach. The Six Standard Autogenic Exercises became a universal form of treatment — designed for greater accessibility. This breaks free from the dependence on the more usual diagnosis and treatment processes with which we are familiar, in favour of a holistic approach involving body, mind and spirit.

The principle is this: it doesn't matter what your symptoms are — use autogenic exercises and tap into your self-healing mechanisms to give yourself a chance to put them right before seeking medical help. Better still: use Autogenic Standard Exercises on a daily basis, keep tapping into your own resources, and, generally, you will prevent ill-health.

A MENTAL EXERCISE DESCRIBED

If you imagine sitting in a chair or lying on a bed in a comfortable, symmetrical manner with your eyes closed, you will already have the picture of what someone practising an AT exercise looks like.

The exercises are easily-learned silent formulae related to the body in a relaxed state. They begin with phrases suggesting heaviness and warmth in the limbs (Standard Exercises 1 and 2), followed by passive focusing on the heartbeat, breathing, abdominal warmth and cool forehead (SEs 3–6).

These exercises usually bring about profound physical relaxation and a state of inner peace and calm. Repetition of the formulae induces a switching off of the body's stress responses. A variety of changes in physical function and brain-wave activity can be measured during autogenic practice, showing that a normalising process takes place (see Chapter 7). This allows the mind/body system to tap into its own self-curative processes.

The technique is often described as 'a meditation suitable for westernised cultures'. The exercises require little expenditure of time, use straightforward language, follow a logical progression and do not rely on any pre-existing belief patterns.

Once learned, they can be used at any time and almost anywhere: on the train or plane, in the office, as a car passenger, or in bed. Short bursts of the exercise can be used to calm you down instantly if you are agitated or in pain.

There are even partial exercises you can use while engaged in any activity, which can keep you calm and stop an unwanted stress response. This might be when standing in a queue, 'white-knuckled' at traffic-lights, on the phone or before answering it, in difficult meetings, or in any other stressful situation

There are no cultural or religious roots to the training, which makes it acceptable to people of any spiritual persuasion, or ethnic origin.

TRAINING OR THERAPY?

Autogenic Therapy is sometimes referred to as Autogenic Training. You are trained to use the exercises by the therapist who guides you through the process of change, which results in a therapeutic outcome. Clients gradually train themselves to tap into and trust their own innate healing capacity, to bring about improved physical and psychological health. Over eight or nine weeks, the whole programme is built up. Each week's exercise forms an integral part of the final whole, and needs to be practised in readiness for the next step.

Once trained, you will have at your fingertips a truly unique healing method that restores balance — moving the system towards homeostasis (see Chapter 7). Many people describe AT as a tool kit for dealing with the stresses and strains of life.

Figure 1: The Benefits of Autogenic Therapy

Increased	Decreased
Good health and resistance to disease	Anxiety
	Panic attacks
Emotional stability	Irritability
Coping ability	Frustration
Well-being	Arguments
Quality of sleep	Cynicism
Ability to relax	Reactions to stress
Self control	Physical symptoms
Peace of mind	Muscular tension
Confidence	Susceptibility to infections and illness
Energy	
Performance at work/sport	Recovery time from illness or injury
Awareness of own needs	
Decision-making skills	Bad dreams
Ability to assert oneself	Need for unhealthy support, caffeine, alcohol, cigarettes or self-medication.
Tolerance of stress	
Calmness	
Ability to relate positively to others	Eating problems
	Anti-social behaviour
Enjoyment of life	Nervous mannerisms
Creativity	

WHO CAN BENEFIT FROM AUTOGENIC THERAPY?

AT has a very wide application in healthcare — see Figure 1. It can be used as part of a comprehensive self-development programme; it can increase creativity, helping writers, artists, musicians and actors. AT often improves performance in sport, enabling many people to achieve their full potential in a diversity of areas. AT is often taught in industry, with great effect as a stress-proofing technique, and for improving interpersonal relationships; or it can help prior to embarking upon a challenging episode in life.

It has been used in every walk of life: from priests and teachers to parents and policemen. It has helped a contestant on a challenging TV contest, as well as Olympic athletes and mountaineers.

THE BENEFITS OF AUTOGENIC THERAPY
Significant improvement can occur within a few weeks. People who have learned AT commonly report results such as those indicated in Figure 1.

WHAT PEOPLE SAY ABOUT AUTOGENIC THERAPY
It is not unusual for people to report that AT has changed their life, which may seem too sweeping a statement to believe. For these people, AT has brought a new awareness of possibilities and choices in the way they conduct their lives. If they feel better mentally, they are very likely to feel better physically. This knowledge gives them confidence and a sense of control over their health and well-being. Here are some comments made by people who have learned AT:

> Autogenic Therapy has given me greater confidence and awareness, a sense of more choice in life. Life is now more positive and pleasurable.
>
> MH, 1996
>
> I am able to relax and deal with daily events. I am more confident and optimistic about the future.
>
> KK, 1997
>
> I feel Autogenic Therapy has helped me more than anything else with my anxiety: very impressed.
>
> JA, 1997
>
> The main change is an improvement in my eczema. I have tried many things but Autogenic Therapy definitely makes my skin healthier, less inflated and less dry.
>
> PW, 1996

I am now able to face public speaking without a tranquilliser.

CC, 1997

I have been able to come off my blood-pressure tablets.

RH, 1996

I feel I now have the tools to cope with life.

CP, 1996

Since learning Autogenic Therapy I am more relaxed in my approach to everything. I am less hurried and putting less pressure on myself. I am not worrying constantly about issues and problems.

LB, 1996

I am getting to sleep faster than I ever have before. I wake properly rested.

BB, 1998

Figure 2: Some Conditions and Problems Helped by Autogenic Therapy

Anger	Loss of creativity migraine
Anxiety	Muscular pain and tension
Arthritis	Negativity
Asthma	Pain
Backache	Palpitations
Bladder disorders	Panic attacks
Bowel problems (Irritable bowel, Colitis)	Pent-up aggression
	Phobias
Chest pains	Physical tension
Circulation problems	Poor circulation
Depression	Pre-menstrual tension
Fatigue	Raised blood pressure
Headaches	Sexual dysfunction
Inability to relax	Skin problems
Lack of confidence	Sleep problems

WHERE CAN YOU FIND AT?

Autogenic therapists work in many different areas, including the following:

- Homoeopathic hospitals
- Homoeopathic practices
- Complementary therapy centres
- Cardiac units
- Hospices
- Psychiatric units
- Psychotherapy practices
- Counselling practices
- Private practice
- GP practices
- Education
- Sports clinics
- Industry
- Occupational health
- Occupational therapy
- Performing arts.

LEARNING AT

It is necessary to learn AT with a qualified practitioner. The exercises are simple to understand, logical and straightforward. They do, however, need to be carried out precisely, and frequent repetition is essential to the learning process.

Initially, an individual interview is conducted to assess the suitability of AT, and the individual needs of the client. The standard exercises are built up gradually over an eight- or nine-session course.

The mind is focused inward, away from external matters, passively observing the effects of the exercise. Dominant left-brain processes are suspended, and the system is allowed to move towards homeostasis (see Chapter 7).

You will learn how to quieten a busy mind to enable passive focus on the body, using a comfortable posture. You will be taught how to focus on repetition of the autogenic formulae, rather than worry about results. You will learn how to recognise autogenic discharges, and deal with resistance. You will be taught to use Intentional Off-loading Exercises to deal with emerging feelings and enhance the process (see Chapter 5). Most important, you will gradually become more aware of yourself as your process unfolds, developing your own strategies for taking control of your life and health.

Personal Adaptation
The Autogenic Standard Exercises can be adapted to include personalised formulae to help with specific goals in performance, motivation or healing.

Timing of a Course
If you suffer from a chronic condition, it is always best to start a course in a quiet phase or before problems get too bad. If possible, try to arrange to learn AT at a time when not too much else is going on in your life. Going on holiday in the middle of an AT course can cause more disruption than you realise. You might think you will have more opportunity to practise your autogenic exercises, but often the result is a disappointment, as your routine is thrown out, and you are constantly in the company of others. It is best to be in your usual routine.

However, if we are too stringent about this, you will never find the right time to start a course. Sometimes the only choice is to 'go for it' — it is amazing how the system can adapt, even when it seems that everything is set against it.

WILL I HAVE TO MAKE ANY LIFE CHANGES?

Changes in your way of operating and reacting do occur, and lifestyle adjustments are sometimes the result. If your lifestyle is the cause of your problems, a realisation that change is needed, and the energy to make those changes, may be a positive outcome of your autogenic process.

Sometimes loved ones around us are unprepared for the changes that AT can bring about. Even when these changes are positive — such as someone becoming more assertive — their unfamiliarity can feel quite unsettling at first. Things will soon settle down as re-adjustment takes place, and relationships can then develop and grow.

The combination of using a deep-relaxation programme, with the added dimension of emotional release when required, gives an individual a remarkable tool-kit for maintaining emotional and physical equilibrium for the rest of their lives.

Once learned, AT is an important and invaluable life skill, providing the inner resources to maintain healthy balance and to deal with stress in body and mind.

CHAPTER 2

PREPARING TO LEARN AUTOGENIC THERAPY (AT)

WHY LEARN WITH A THERAPIST?

'Why do I have to learn AT with a therapist, when I have seen it in books and articles in teach-yourself form? AT is always put forward as a simple technique, so why not? Is it so difficult?'

The trouble with the written word is that it is all you have. There is no guide or personal support — no one to help you with queries, or to give you reassurance or back-up when you are in doubt. You could give up at the first hurdle. You need a knowledgeable therapist who will monitor your practice and give you feedback on your progress. Although the technique itself is very easy, the responses to training are endlessly varied and unique to you.

For most people the AT course is relatively smooth and easy-going, with any 'blips' working themselves through. However, the autogenic process does allow emerging material to rise to the surface — this needs release. Without good support at each stage, at best it is unlikely that you would progress much further than simple relaxation, 'ploughing through' the course on a superficial level, and missing out on all the subtleties of process and change. At worst, you might find yourself experiencing an uncomfortable response which could cause you to give up. You would then miss the opportunity to understand and work through your all-important re-adjustment process, which leads you to the enormous benefits to be gained from AT.

MONITORING PROGRESS

The therapist, knowing your background, will be able to help you to proceed in a way that keeps the process comfortable — slowing it down if necessary. Some people will need to spend longer on one part of the course, while, for others, less time might be required, depending on the response to any particular formula.

EXPLANATIONS AND DEMONSTRATIONS

The therapist will explain the rationale for each formula, with clear guidelines. There is always the opportunity to ask questions. Then the exercise will be demonstrated and practised. Immediate feedback often brings to light some misunderstandings or anxieties, and these can be dealt with on the spot.

Errors can be picked up and minor adjustments suggested. These small corrections can make a big difference to the individual response to an exercise. Discussion about home practice environment and lifestyle issues will also contribute to the general support, so that you understand the optimum conditions for the best progress. Sometimes this is about the general approach — for example, whether or not you explain to the family what you are doing.

MOTIVATION

Regular attendance at a course will help you to keep motivated to practise. You will report back each week, using a training diary in which you have recorded your observations. There is lots of reassurance as you see others progress, while sharing the training difficulties with people who are at the same stage as you.

MANAGING FEEDBACK

Sometimes reactions to the exercises can feel worrying. For example, a symptom which reminds you of a past illness can occur fleetingly, or linger for a few hours after the exercise. You may perceive this as a problem, and your therapist, after careful questioning, will help you by explaining the process, and will encourage you to allow it. You will receive reassurance that your responses are normal.

SUPPORT IS ALWAYS AVAILABLE

Sometimes it is necessary to clarify something with your therapist between sessions. If you find yourself encountering difficulties which get in the way of your AT practice, you can discuss this. It is important to keep up the flow of the course, as each exercise (formula) prepares you for the next one.

MODIFICATIONS

The Six Standard Exercises have been devised and developed and have stood the test of time. In themselves, they seem quite innocuous, but the fascination of AT lies in the response each individual makes. So it is possible, and sometimes necessary, to change the timing, wording or order of some formulae so that the process can be reduced or slowed down a little.

Now — do you still want to learn AT from a book?

FINDING A QUALIFIED AUTOGENIC THERAPIST

In the UK and Ireland, the British Autogenic Society is the only professional organisation which trains autogenic therapists. BAS-trained therapists will have professional insurance, and they are likely to be under regular supervision and be undergoing continuing professional development.

QUESTIONS FOR YOUR PROSPECTIVE BAS THERAPIST

- Cost of the courses and methods of payment?
- Do they take groups or individuals?
- Dates and venue of the courses?
- Will your information be kept confidential?
- Is the therapist available between sessions?
- What size are the groups? (Maximum 8 or 10)

YOUR RELATIONSHIP WITH THE THERAPIST

The therapist may be highly qualified, but it is important that you have a good therapeutic relationship with them. From your initial phone conversation, you will have a feeling about the person. There is nothing to stop you shopping around, talking to several therapists if you have a choice in your area. They should provide you with good information, and be clear about their style of practice. All BAS therapists will have gone through their own AT process before starting therapist training.

Ask yourself what you feel about this person. Could you share intimate details with them? Are they approachable? Would you feel happy to phone them if you had a query?

PRE-COURSE ASSESSMENT

This initial consultation is the starting point of your journey with AT, and the first task is to complete a comprehensive questionnaire. You will meet your therapist individually, discuss the issues around your reasons for joining a course, and the processes involved. It is important to discuss any existing medical or psychological condition, as the autogenic process might affect it. Your past history and current state of health and social circumstances are all relevant.

As in most effective complementary therapies, it is recognised that as you begin to tap into your self-righting mechanisms, symptoms can appear to get worse before they get better. Your therapist will explain the principles of the autogenic philosophy and how the process might unfold. The assessment will leave you a little more knowledgeable and eager to get started.

It is likely that you will explore the implications of:

- Past issues which have left an effect on your health
- What you will have to put into your training to get the best out of it
- Current health issues which may need monitoring or investigating
- How AT may help you (no promise will be made as to outcome)
- Whether AT is the right thing for you to be doing
- Whether it is the right time to be doing it
- If not AT, what else might be suitable.

All questionnaires will cover:

- Your physical health — past and present
- Any prescribed medication
- The use of non-prescribed drugs — as a habit or experimentally: whether you had unpleasant experiences with these
- Whether you have spent time in hospital, and any associated unpleasant experiences
- Women will complete their gynaecological and obstetric history
- Family health — parents and siblings
- Your own birth — it is the first traumatic event we have all gone through and will carry memory on some level
- Accidents and injuries
- Childhood and development
- Whether you have experienced altered states of consciousness through various triggers, e.g. hypnosis, alcohol, overdose, chemical fumes
- Whether you have suffered emotional disturbance — e.g. agitation, depression, panic attacks, feelings of loss of own reality, suicidal feelings
- General health and lifestyle questions. These are subjective: how you feel in the present.

Questions about your family health and family status will help your therapist to see what support systems you have or, perhaps, what support you have to give to your family.

Completing the form takes some time, and doing so is *the first step in looking at yourself.* You will bring the form to your appointment, and a discussion is held alongside it. The time this takes will vary according to the setting in which you are learning AT. It is usually an hour or less, but in some instances may need longer, or two consultations. All of this is, of course, completely confidential. The more honest and open you can be, the better.

Your therapist will want to make sure that you are a self-motivated person, and willing to put in the required effort to get the most out of the course. You will need to ensure that you have time and space to devote to yourself during the training period and that you have some internal and external support on your journey.

Don't be daunted by the thoroughness of this assessment. Many people find that this opportunity to review their life and health actually begins their process of change. We are often told: 'I feel so much better already.' The brain seems to appreciate that you have made a decision to help yourself, and you have made a start.

Stress Load
Sometimes it is clear that a client may be 'heavily loaded'. This does not necessarily mean that AT is not recommended for them. For example, if the client had a disturbed upbringing, and their parents and whole family might have been subjected to an acrimonious divorce, it may be evident that the client is holding on to painful feelings from that time. Awareness is raised at this point, and the therapist will be assessing what modifications it may be necessary to make during the course.

CONTRA-INDICATIONS

For a large majority of people, Autogenic Therapy is absolutely safe, and there is no reason why they shouldn't learn it and make it an integral part of their lives.

However, there are a few circumstances when it is not recommended. These circumstances are known as *contra-indications*. Schultz and Luthe described two categories of contra-indication which give a baseline of awareness to the therapist.

ABSOLUTE CONTRA-INDICATIONS
There are some people for whom AT is not suitable. These include:

1   Anyone suffering from a psychotic illness such as schizophrenia or manic depression (bi-polar condition); in these cases AT might trigger a psychotic response. (In some circumstances, such as under close supervision in a psychiatric in-patient unit, modified AT might be used.)
2   Those with severe learning difficulties
3   Children under the age of five.

In the latter situations, they would be unable to understand the tasks or explain their responses.

RELATIVE CONTRA-INDICATIONS

There are circumstances where the standard course might need adapting to accommodate various symptoms or situations.

1. Children Over the Age of Five

A shortened course can be used. We would recommend that at least one of the parents should learn AT for themselves, as this would be the best support they could give their child.

2. Learning Difficulties

Here, learning AT would be at the discretion of the therapist and the person's carer. An individually tailored course, depending on the level of understanding and support available, is essential.

3. Physical Conditions

If someone is experiencing serious physical symptoms that have not been investigated or diagnosed, or if they suffer from an illness that is not being monitored, it would be unwise to proceed with AT. We would insist that they consult their GP or other specialist before starting a course.

If there is an unstable condition, such as recent heart attack or stroke, it is unwise to start an AT course until at least three months have elapsed.

4. Psychological Disturbance

Depression can occur in cycles, such as SAD (Seasonal Affective Disorder). In this case, it might be best to learn AT during a good phase, and build on that, rather than embark on autogenic work in a low phase, as it might cause more, if temporary, disturbance.

5. Substance Addiction/Abuse

Anyone who has recently been using non-prescribed mind-altering substances may be unsuitable to learn AT. They could be unreliable and erratic in their approach, and could encounter flashbacks of recent 'bad trips'. All of this might well put the client off, and it creates difficulties for the therapist in monitoring the process. However, when there is evidence of determined efforts at withdrawing from using these substances, or the person has been 'clean' for several months, AT can be very useful as part of rehabilitation.

Someone suffering from alcoholism would need to have been in recovery for at least six months and have good motivation and support.

COMMUNICATION/LANGUAGE DIFFICULTIES

It would be unwise to proceed if there were problems with communication because of language differences or lack of contact with the client. Reporting back the response to the exercises is essential if the full potential of the training is to be realised and difficulties avoided.

LACK OF MOTIVATION

Learning AT is a serious commitment, and good results will be gained only if the course is conscientiously followed all the way through. It would be unwise to embark on a course unless you are motivated to work on yourself with a reasonable insight into your own processes. If you are going to give up if things get uncomfortable, and are not willing to go back to your therapist to sort out any difficulties, you will not get the best out of the course, and might lay yourself open to unresolved problems.

AT is Not Crisis Management

Careful consideration needs to be given to doing the course at the right time. Mid-crisis is not, perhaps, the best time to embark upon a challenging nine-week course. Sometimes a little first-aid in the form of short-term medication or counselling can help to calm things down before starting an AT course. An example of this might be when a close bereavement has recently occurred.

Summary

Therapists will use their discretion in all the above scenarios of relative contra-indications.

AT Alongside Other Medical Treatment

As AT is a non-drug, non-invasive method, it is often used as a support to other treatments, whether conventional or complementary. When the mind and body are in the habit of switching on their relaxation/recovery mode, the effect of other interventions is usually enhanced. So, the aromatherapy massage/reflexology treatment, or antibiotics, are received into the system more quickly and efficiently than without AT. In this case, it is important to have good communication between the different treatment agencies.

Other Therapies During Training

Although AT works well alongside other therapies, the authors always suggest that, if possible, new treatment is not started at the same time as learning AT, in order to observe clearly the autogenic process.

The Role of the Client

A course in Autogenic Training requires you to do all the work to bring about change in yourself. You will get out of it what you put into it, so you will need to follow instructions. The sooner you get into a routine of practice (three to four times per day), the easier you will find it. Note the times of day where your AT exercises feel most rewarding, and use them as a gift to yourself. Find out how 'less-than-perfect' exercises feel — all exercises are valid. Those who perceive early results are those who pay attention to detail. Here are some ideas to keep in mind.

- Keep all your AT documents together in a file.
- Always complete your diary and remember to take it with you to every training session.
- Complete any charts or inventories you are given.
- Practise regularly in the best environment available.
- Tell people at home that you need peace and quiet for your exercises.
- Put pets out of the room.
- Practise the Standard Exercises three or four times a day.
- Do not change the wording of formulae or invent your own.
- Make sure that you use the postures correctly.
- Use short-stitch when appropriate (see chapter 3).
- Make time for off-loading (Intentional) exercises.
- Let your therapist know if you have any disturbing reactions.
- Let your therapist know if you do not understand any aspect of the instructions.
- Let your therapist know if things are improving.
- Make a note of any general queries you might have for the next session.
- Tell your therapist if you are receiving any other treatment.
- Tell your therapist if you start taking any drugs, or if the dose of those you are taking changes.
- Tell your therapist in good time if you are going to miss a session.
- If you have missed a session, you should arrange to catch up before the next one.

If you feel, during the course, that AT is not for you, talk to your therapist if you want to leave the course before the end. It is to be hoped that the discussion will bring to the fore that you are well into your AT process, and that to keep going is better that leaving it unfinished. If circumstances are such that it is agreed that you should not complete, things need to be rounded off safely, so that you will still gain from the experience so far.

TIME FOR THE PROCESS

Autogenic Therapy is usually learned over a period of three to four months. This comprises:

* The initial consultation/assessment
* An eight- or nine-week course in consecutive weeks
* A follow-up session six to eight weeks after the final session.

The learning time-scale is very important, in order to allow gradual assimilation of each of the autogenic exercises. The introduction of the Six Standard Exercises is carefully planned in a weekly progression, which allows your unique self-righting system to do its work. Each new autogenic formula is incorporated into the preceding week's exercise, giving a structured, yet continuous, flow of practice. During the course, there is time for practice, feedback, adaptation, if necessary, and general monitoring of the process.

Each autogenic exercise has the potential, when first used, to bring about a strong response: either some kind of resistance, or the need to off-load emerging feelings. It is important that the process is kept moving, and it may be a mistake to stay too long focused on a particular exercise.

In some circumstances it is possible to learn AT in a shorter period, or perhaps split the course into two parts (five sessions, a break, then the last four sessions). This might suit people who travel a lot, or university students who are not resident in one area long enough to complete nine consecutive weeks.

Think of the time it takes for a broken bone to recover: about six weeks. Any recovery process involving the miracles of the human body and mind must be given time. We are always suspicious (indeed, concerned about safety) when we hear of someone claiming to have learned AT at a weekend workshop. Where is the time for the process?

Over the learning period, the exercises are gradually assimilated into an 'autogenic whole'. In the beginning, frequent repetition of the exercise is required, to instigate your process of change. Full assimilation may take several weeks and is always spontaneous. Maybe we can never quite define it, but we gradually become aware of a sense of wholeness and inner well-being.

WHAT KIND OF COURSE — GROUP OR INDIVIDUAL?

It is possible to learn AT on your own as an individual client, or in a small group. Both ways have their advantages, although not all therapists offer both.

GROUP
If you join a group, there could be any number between three and eight in it. At the very most you might be in a class of ten.

'The Closed Group'
Confidentiality
The group setting is always a confidential one. You will be expected not to reveal or discuss outside the group things you hear about other group members. It is up to you what you may wish to reveal/discuss about yourself in the group. Your personal inform-ation will be kept confidential, and you will have access to your therapist outside the group should any confidential matter arise.

Start Together
The group starts and finishes the course at the same time. It would be quite inappropriate for members of the group to be at differ-ent stages of the course.

Advantages of Learning AT in a Group
You will find that you are not alone, and whatever is going on for you in your autogenic process, the likelihood is that others will be

having similar experiences. Other group members will ask questions of the therapist, so this extra information will inevitably increase your understanding of AT. There is support from the other members in overcoming any practical difficulties, and there is acknowledgement of your efforts — both of which help to encourage you to *trust* in your healing and self-righting processes.

It's more fun in a group! There are aspects of camaraderie and friendship which will make you look forward to each weekly session — if for no other reason than that you are curious to know how everyone else is doing.

Cost

Learning AT in a group is usually much cheaper than learning it individually.

INDIVIDUAL

Advantages

There is time for more confidential discussion during the sessions. Timing can be flexible, such as when a regular weekly meeting is not possible because of a client's working patterns. If adjustment of the regular course is necessary, this can be managed with real individual flexibility.

CAN I START AS AN INDIVIDUAL AND THEN JOIN A GROUP?

This is not usually recommended, for timing reasons. Very occasionally, it may be necessary to exit from a group and continue individually, but the need for this would be assessed depending on what material emerges.

THE LEARNING ENVIRONMENT

AT is an easy method of switching off the stress response, and we always recommend that you practise anywhere: on the bus; in a train; at the station; on the beach; in a rehearsal room; in the passenger seat of a car; in an airport lounge while waiting for your (delayed) flight; at your desk; in the loo at work. You will surprise yourself, after a little practice, when you discover how easily you can 'switch off', despite noise or bright light. It is as though you can enjoy a mini-holiday or retreat by going into yourself for a few minutes to 'recharge your batteries'.

However, at the start of your AT course, when you are new to it, you will need to be a little more careful about your learning environment. In the first few weeks, interruptions from the environment can feel very frustrating, as the 'autogenic state' is quite fragile, sensitive and easily disturbed. Even the ticking of a clock can become a major distraction.

If you can, practise alone in the beginning. If other people are around you, especially at home or at work, you may feel a sense of being 'on duty', which is quite inhibiting and might not allow a complete switch-off. You will enjoy the exercises if you have created a place of freedom for yourself, and the reward will be a sense of making good progress.

NOISE

Early on, one of the greatest distractions can be background noise: traffic, ticking clocks, humming or clicking radiators and fridges, air-craft noise. You will soon learn how to pay attention to these noises (or even the possibility of noise) before you begin an exercise. Simply acknowledging sound, and accepting it, is often the way to reduce the significance of the sound, allowing us to 'leave it alone'.

Sudden noise which occurs during the exercise may shock you at first. Eventually, you will learn that when someone bangs a door, there is no need to react and let it interrupt you.

INTERRUPTIONS

The phone; cries of 'Mum, where are you?'; 'Where's my …?'; the doorbell; your boss demanding an instant meeting; your neighbour 'just popping in'— sometimes it seems as though the world is con-spiring against you simply to sabotage your autogenic exercises. You know what you are trying to do and, in spite of the best will in the world, you seem unable to do it.

Unplug or switch off the phone; ignore the doorbell. It will feel hard at first, but you might even miss the double-glazing salesman!

Sometimes our training is as much about educating others as it is about educating ourselves. *You* know what you want to do, but does anyone else? Can you ask for ten minutes' peace and quiet? Does your family know that if they call you and you do not respond, you are doing an exercise and, if left alone, will reappear shortly, relaxed and refreshed?

Jane remembers a story from her own experience:

My youngest son was two years old when I first learned AT and would join in my 'thinking exercise' with me. One day, when he was four, he needed me urgently. I heard his footsteps at the door of the room, and a few exasperated breaths to see if I would react. I did not want him to learn that he could interrupt me whenever he chose, so I stopped using the autogenic formulae, held my posture and kept my eyes closed. In this instance, I was training him, even though the actual exercise was abandoned.

Next, a hot whisper in my left ear: 'Mummy — can I have my pocket money?'

Much as I wanted to give him a big hug, I stayed still, eyes closed. I whispered back: 'Yes — in a minute, when I'm ready.'

'Thank you.'

He was quite happy with this, and, far from being frustrated by the interruption, I was proud of his sensitivity, later giving him a big hug and his cash.

Telling the Family

When telling the people around you, you will not be describing AT in detail. But, whatever your circumstances, it is better both for you and for your family if no one is taken by surprise — and you will have to prepare the ground.

If Jane's son had not known that she often sits in a chair with her eyes closed, he might have become alarmed. As it was, he did his best to be as gentle as he could. So Jane acknowledged him, while still keeping the boundary of her own space.

Fire! Reassurance

It's OK. If the house is on fire, you *will* realise, and the correct stress response *will* kick in, and you *will* be able to close your exercise instantly and deal with the emergency. The beauty of AT is that all your responses are normal. You do not 'leave' your immediate surroundings.

LIGHT

If the light is too strong, it may, at first, be distracting. A dim light is preferred, or you could turn your back on the source of light. If you are practising before sleep, you will be in the dark — that's fine too.

TEMPERATURE

Try and organise a setting with an even temperature. Too warm or too cold will interfere with your comfort, and also with your concentration.

PHYSICAL DISCOMFORT

You need to feel comfortable in your body before you start. A full bladder or tight clothing will distract you and demand all your attention. Always loosen tight clothing if you can — and remove your shoes if you are in private.

POSTURE

There are three postures which have been specifically designed to minimise any distraction from the body during practice. These are described in more detail in Chapter 3. You might use an armchair; any dining-type chair, or a stool; or you might lie on a floor, or in bed before sleep.

All the postures are designed to create a symmetry in the trunk and limbs, with the muscles in a neutral rest position, halfway between their full range of movement. This helps the concentration to be at its most effective, and allows practice anywhere.

CONTINUING PRACTICE

Sometimes we cannot find 'ideal' conditions. Do the best you can, with whatever is available. In time, you will find that it doesn't matter.

Example

One man was visiting friends and found himself sleeping in an attic room with an irritating hissing cistern. His heart sank: 'How am I supposed to do my AT with that'? He got into bed, and amazed himself by reaching a deep level of meditation very quickly with AT. He said that the hissing sound even helped him — a constant in the background which enhanced his focus.

SUMMARY

It is important when learning AT that stimuli around you are reduced as far as possible, thus avoiding interference with, or distraction from, your inner processes.

ACTIVE AND PASSIVE CONCENTRATION

ACTIVE CONCENTRATION

When we concentrate on a task, we are usually striving to achieve a result — some sort of goal. The activity is governed by the end result, and requires specific attention: how the task is carried out; using learned skills in doing it; regarding it critically; correcting mistakes; doing it as best we can; taking pride in it. The brain is engaged in receiving and processing input from the world around — external to us.

This type of activity stems from the left hemisphere of the brain (see Chapter 10), which is associated with intellectual pursuits, learning new skills, attention to detail. We are used to striving when we put the left hemisphere to work. Think how we struggled to learn to tie our shoelaces, or read Ladybird books; how difficult it was to manage first and second gears when we learned to drive! And marvel at the way our brains have converted those difficulties into automatic responses. (Prove it to yourself now by tying laces slowly, identifying every move, and writing down each instruction as you go. It is very difficult to unravel an automatic response once it is in place.) This is Active Concentration.

PASSIVE CONCENTRATION

Now we are in the opposite realm. When we are passive, we let go of all the associations of Active Concentration: we use no learned skills, there is no critical judgement, there is no concern about result or 'doing it well', and no correction of mistakes. Most important — there is no goal, no striving to achieve.

The right hemisphere of the brain is engaged in responding to, and automatically processing, material from the internal world. During an autogenic exercise, this phase of brain activity is often described as 'the autogenic state'.

Encouraging Passive Concentration

You will learn how to take your attention inward, and focus on various parts of the body, relating to each Standard Exercise. The very fact that you will close your eyes to practise means that your focus will change — from looking out, to looking inwards.

Gradually you will become more aware of your body (a new focus is introduced each week), and you will become aware of any sensations present. It is as counter-productive to try and produce or enhance these sensations as it is to try and suppress them. The task is simply to accept them, without judgement. Some will feel more pleasant than others, but all these internal sensations are part of the healing blue-print which is unique to you. You are learning to tap into this process of self-adjustment, with passive acceptance.

Physical characteristics of Passive Concentration

* Slack jaw
* Relaxed face

- General feeling of relaxation
- Increased salivation — swallowing or dribbling
- Borborygmi (tummy rumbles)
- Slower pulse
- Slower breathing
- Muscle twitching, indicating release of tension (the autogenic discharge)
- Random thoughts or memories

PASSIVE AWARENESS

In your first session of the AT course, the principles of Passive Concentration will be explained, and you will be encouraged to be the Passive Observer. These are attitudes of mind which you will adopt during the exercises, which allow the process to occur unimpeded. Our usual goal-setting and striving attitudes are set aside, and any phenomena are simply observed. This is Passive Awareness.

As your therapist leads you through your very first exercise, you may find yourself worrying that you are not doing it right. You *are* doing it right, except for one thing — *thinking that you are doing it wrong!* We are not used to 'doing' or 'learning' anything which is not measured by results, so we can feel uneasy just letting be. But critical judgement about the quality of the exercise will spoil it by impeding the brain's natural processes. It is not necessary to do an exercise 'better than the last' or even 'as good as the last'. No active effort is necessary when you do AT. It is non-competitive, there are no active goals, and it makes us more than usually aware of the mind and the body.

SUMMARY

Creating a good environment, ensuring a comfortable neutral posture, and silent repetition of the training formulae all encourage the switch to a 'Passive Concentration state'. Regular practice enables you to switch into this state at will, and stay there for increasing periods of time. *AT is so easy to do, at first it can feel really difficult.*

CHAPTER 3

A TEN-SESSION AUTOGENIC THERAPY COURSE

*W*e would remind you that it is not recommended that you attempt to learn AT without the help of a professionally trained therapist. Your collaboration with them is essential for the optimum results from your Autogenic Training.

Although we will describe here a group process, remember that AT is also frequently taught individually.

THE FIRST SESSION

The first session will include the following:

- An optional written exercise reflecting on the question, 'Why am I here?' — for your eyes only
- Management of the group — procedures and ground rules
- Introductions
- Introductory background to AT and its philosophy
- Discussion of practice environment
- Discussion of the importance of daily practice, which prepares you for the next week's step
- Demonstration and practice of the training postures
- The body check/scan as a preparation for an exercise
- The closure (or 'cancel') of the exercise
- Introduction to the concept of the Passive Observer
- Discussion on the use of Passive Concentration
- Discussion of the Training Diary — its importance to your progress

- The week's exercise: Short Stitch and/or Standard Exercise 1 (Heaviness).

WRITTEN EXERCISE — FIRST PART

This exercise is a very useful starting point — a simple personal assessment of progress. A period of nine weeks is not a long time in anyone's life, but when engaged in a profound process of physical and psychological change, the memory is surprisingly short. So, on Day 1, capture on paper your thoughts about why you wish to learn AT.

The group sits with this task for about ten minutes, everyone writing their answers to the questions: 'Why am I here?' 'What do I want from AT?' 'What are my current complaints?' 'What are my wishes for the future?' In addition, it is useful to write a self-portrait, 'Me in My Life Now', about your life at home and at work, your health, relationships, hobbies, fun, etc.

Doing this plays a significant part in your process. Clients invariably say, at the second part of the exercise (when re-reading later on): 'This is fascinating. I'd forgotten how I felt back then.'

All the sheets of paper are labelled with the name of their owner, and sealed in an envelope, which is kept by the therapist until the ninth session, or perhaps the follow-up session. Then they are returned, after you have written a second sheet. This time: 'Where am I now? What has AT done for me so far?' You may well be surprised at the differences, some of them quite subtle.

INTRODUCTIONS

The group members introduce themselves, using first names only, and saying a little about themselves if they wish. You may feel reassured that these are ordinary people just like yourself, and that they, like you, are looking for ways to help themselves.

INTRODUCTORY BACKGROUND TO AT AND ITS PHILOSOPHY

Your therapist will probably introduce several aspects of this at various times during the course (see Chapter 10).

THE TRAINING POSTURES

These are illustrated in Figure 3. In your first AT session you will be shown these in detail, and how to adopt them. It will also be explained why they are important.

The Purpose of Posture

It is important that AT is practised with the minimum of interference. The recommended postures ensure that the body is able to relax and let go of tension, while being supported. Lingering tension is a distraction and will prevent adequate Passive Concentration. Not only will you need to avoid muscular tension, but also you will need to sit or lie in a position of balance and symmetry. AT is never practised with legs crossed, or arms folded. The brain needs to identify right and left, in order for autogenic processes to unfold, and body parts should not be in contact with each other more than the minimum necessary. As you get used to these postures, you will find how unrewarding it is to do AT when you have been careless about adopting the correct stance.

We do not sit or lie with the palms of the hands uppermost, as is the case in many meditation methods. One reason for this is a matter of comfort: try out the difference now. Place each hand on each thigh palms down, fingers slightly spread but not stretched. You should feel quite comfortable — no jarring. Now turn your palms upwards. You will probably feel a pulling discomfort in the forearms, elbows and near your shoulders. We are looking for a posture that is physically neutral — stretched or contracted muscles are not relaxed.

Another reason for 'palms down' can be acknowledged as the more spiritual side of AT practice. The position of the palms when turned up might be interpreted as opening up to the universe — almost an attitude of supplication, involving processes from without. AT is a contemplative method, looking inwards. 'Palms down' might be the second indicator, alongside closing the eyes, of looking inward.

A variety of postures make AT instantly accessible whatever your circumstances. The whole point of AT is that you have it with you wherever you are. You do not rely on tapes, special clothing, or even much time. Your inner voice is ready always — just tap into it when you can.

When you are learning, the postures should be varied in order to accustom you to their use. The exercises can be done in bed, and, if you should fall asleep during them, you will shift automatically from the autogenic state to normal sleep.

The Simple Sitting Posture (SSP)

This can be used in any upright chair, preferably a traditional dining-room style, with one leg at each corner. In this posture, your body is supported only by the front legs of the chair and your own feet on the floor. Your spine 'slumps' and bends over, allowing a combination of relaxing muscles and also stretching the back and shoulders. This is a good posture for releasing neck and shoulder tension, and, although it can feel unfamiliar and strange at first (mother must have told you never to slouch), the more you use it, the more comfortable it becomes. Many people find it the 'good, working AT posture'. You can even lock yourself into the bathroom and perch on the side of the bath, or use the loo at work.

The Armchair Posture (ACP)

The ACP is the most versatile of the three. You can use it in any style of chair, although, as its name suggests, a comfortable armchair is the most obvious. Here, you will be sitting with your back supported by the chair-back. You might rest your hands beside your legs, on your lap, or on the arms of the chair. Your head can rest on the chair-back, with or without a cushion, or it can balance in a neutral position, reducing the tension in your neck muscles as far as possible. The ACP can be adapted to your situation: in the car (passenger seat only, please), bus or train; in the airport lounge waiting for delayed flights; or on the plane (especially if you are nervous of flying).

The Horizontal Posture (HP)

This one speaks for itself. You will lie on your back, in bed or on the floor. This is most usually used for practising AT as you go to sleep. Your head/neck will be supported with one or two pillows. Your arms and hands will rest comfortably, palms down, beside your body, but not touching it. Your legs will not touch each other, and your feet will probably turn outwards as they relax. Before sleep, as you take up your posture, you will be under your duvet or sheets and blankets. You will make sure that your feet are not squashed by bedclothes, as this can cause discomfort and distraction. If you have any low back pain in this posture, a pillow supporting the knees can relieve it.

Figure 3: Training Postures

1. The Simple Sitting Posture

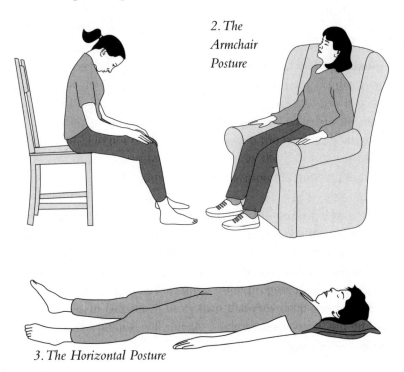

2. The Armchair Posture

3. The Horizontal Posture

Another Posture - the 'Continental Posture'

This posture's name is a mystery to us! However, it is very useful in certain situations. Here, you would sit up on a floor, or in bed, with your feet out in front of you, and your hands resting palms down on your legs, or beside you, which ever is the most comfortable. You would use this if you were in hospital for example, or in your own bed, wanting to practise before you get up in the morning, but reducing the risk of going back to sleep. If you sit on the floor, and lean against a wall, make sure this is not too cold, as this can cause distraction. Use a coat or a cushion to lean on.

THE BODY CHECK/SCAN

Once settled into the correct posture, you need to check that you are ready to start your exercise. A few moments are taken to do a 'mental walk' through the body in preparation, asking yourself: 'Am I sitting comfortably?' Work from the feet, all the way up through your limbs and trunk, through to the jaw. This moves the focus away from the environment and into the body. Obvious tension is let go, or merely observed and allowed, helping the mind and body to settle.

Once the scan is done — taking only twenty to thirty seconds — you will be ready to begin. The body scan is not a relaxation exercise in itself. The very word 'relax' can sometimes set up a resistance ('Relax? Who says?') and impede your concentration.

THE CLOSURE OF THE EXERCISE (CANCEL)

Each exercise has a clear and comforting structure. The 'close' (or cancel, as it is often known) is used to switch the mind out of the autogenic state and return the mind and body to a normal state of alertness — ready for action. It is important that the brain knows the difference between the two states of being. You will learn to make two fists, flex the arms sharply, take a deep breath, and have a good stretch. This restores muscle tone in your limbs. Finally, you will open your eyes, and your mind will return to full alertness, reconnecting with your surroundings.

During an exercise, there is no disconnection with reality. AT does not transport you somewhere else, like a 'trip'. You are always in control, aware of your body in its posture, but the deep relaxation you may experience might make you feel 'miles away'. However, you will always be easily roused should something demand your attention.

In the early days of training, the exercise is practised in a cycle of three repeats, with a close between each one. After each close there is a brief moment to settle back into the posture. Following the third and final close, you will rest for a few moments to contemplate the exercise and acknowledge what you experienced.

Then you will note any sensations in your **training diary** (Chapter 4).

INTRODUCTION TO THE CONCEPT OF THE PASSIVE OBSERVER

We encourage the whole being to 'sit back' and observe the results of any exercise while we practise it. As we use Passive Concentration, we are letting go of active striving. The Passive Observer is your inner witness — the part of you which impartially notes what is going on. The Passive Observer has no care for 'a good result', or whether any response is correct or not. The Passive Observer watches, notes, and *accepts,* without judgement or criticism.

Example

One client, although doing his exercises very regularly, used constantly to berate himself for needing 'to do more work on that' — 'I must try harder'. It took a few weeks for him to realise that all he needed to do was simply to wait for the spontaneous result.

ESTABLISHING MENTAL CONTACT

For the first exercise, we focus on the dominant arm, to introduce the idea of heaviness in it. You will be shown how to make mental contact with the arm. One way of doing this is first to place your left hand on your right shoulder (the reverse if you are left-handed) and run your hand down your arm to the fingertips, and up again, several times. As you do this, you will have three aspects of awareness operating: physical contact (your hand touching your arm); visual contact (watching what you are doing); mental contact (thinking about what you are doing).

Now, close your eyes and continue with the physical and mental contact — you have let go of the visual. Keep your eyes closed, and place your left hand on your left knee, and keep going with the mental contact. You are now resting, with your eyes closed, with mental contact — or focus — on your dominant arm.

Whatever you experience at this stage, *this is Passive Concentration:* simply focusing on the area without influencing it in any way. Once into the exercise, you will repeat the autogenic formula about heaviness in your arm, while adopting the attitude of mind which is the Passive Observer.

PRIMING — INTRODUCING THE SHORT-STITCH EXERCISE

This is a very brief exercise which uses a fragment of the full Heaviness exercise (Standard Exercise 1), allowing frequent and very brief visits to the autogenic state. It lasts no longer than two to three minutes overall. It focuses on the suggestion of heaviness in the dominant arm only, allowing a gentle introduction to the autogenic process. The purpose of this is to train the brain to switch into the autogenic state and maintain passive concentration. There is no time to 'do it wrong'.

The Short-Stitch was given its name by Dr Luthe, as a means to illustrate the concept that AT can be practised little and often, rather than always needing a significant amount of time. There is lots of closure (cancelling) with short-stitch, so at times it can feel quite frustrating. However, it is extremely effective to prepare the way for lengthier exercises.

Each little 'stitch' of exercise lasts about twenty or thirty seconds. It comprises repetition of the formula two or three times, and then closing. Then you will repeat this 'stitch' six or eight times before the final close. Your string of six or eight 'stitches' will complete an autogenic practice session. You might do six or eight (or even ten) of these practice sessions at intervals spread through the day, writing up your observations in your diary after each session. Few achieve this amount, but for those who get near, they will be very well 'into' their autogenic process, and will have plenty to report, often including frustration about the brevity of the exercise!

The many uses of the short–stitch exercise are discussed in Chapter 4. At this point, it is used to train passive concentration.

Practice of Short-Stitch in the Group
This is done in all the three postures if possible. After each exercise, the group gives verbal feedback. This is helpful to all. The therapist can pick up on any difficulties or errors. Each group member listens to the others, which will enhance their own experience.

From the second session, the pattern of the session is set in place. It will go something like this:

• *Practice of Previous Week's Exercise — Revision*
  This is a good way to start the session. It reminds everyone of what they have been (or should have been) doing. Sometimes it is a surprise to find how slowly the therapist talks them through. This is a good reminder and 'brings people back' to what it is all about.
• *Go-round / Feedback on the Week's Practice*
• *A Review of Postures to Correct any Errors*
• *The Introduction of the Next Autogenic Formula*
• *The Practice of the New Exercise*
• *Verbal Feedback after Each Practice*
• *Other Relevant Discussion Topics*

THE SECOND SESSION
INTRODUCTION OF HEAVINESS (STANDARD EXERCISE 1)
PART ONE

PRACTICE OF SHORT-STITCH
GO-ROUND/FEEDBACK ON LAST WEEK
This is primarily verbal. Each person has their turn to describe their week's practice of AT. The therapist will read each diary,

make comments, correct any errors of practice, and generally support what you have been doing.

INTRODUCE THE FIRST STANDARD EXERCISE (SE1)

This exercise uses suggestions (formulae) about Heaviness in all the limbs, e.g. 'My arm is heavy', etc.

Rationale and Theory of 'Heaviness'

In the early days of research into the physiological effects of deep relaxation, hypnosis and sleep, the most common report was a feeling of heaviness and warmth in the limbs. Schultz used this as the foundation for what became Autogenic Training, and Heaviness became the first of his Six Standard Autogenic Exercises.

The heaviness formulae focus on each limb in turn, using the same attitude of passive concentration as in short-stitch. As tension is released from the muscles, so the weight of the limb is experienced.

Practice of the Heaviness Exercise

The therapist leads the group through the new exercise, using the various postures, with feedback after each practice. At the end of the session, the group may well practise the new exercise silently, using the 'autogenic inner voice'. It may be evident at this stage that, although some feedback from the limbs may have been observed, it will not necessarily be perceived as heaviness, but as lightness, tingling, fullness, etc. This is perfectly normal and, as long as the feelings have not been disturbing, they should be accepted with passive observation. A few people may never experience a feeling of heaviness.

THE WEEK'S PRACTICE PATTERN

You are asked to practise this exercise at home in a pattern which is set up for the rest of the course. This is easy to remember because everything goes in 'threes'.

- Set up your day so you can do three (or four) AT sessions.
- Choose one of the three postures for each session.
- In any one session, practise three exercises (closing each exercise as you go).
- In any one exercise, each autogenic formula is repeated three times.

Whatever exercise you are working on in a given week, the practice regime is the same. We often refer to this as '3x3' — that is, three sessions per day, with three exercises in each session.

The time this takes is going to vary according to the stage of the course you are at. The full heaviness exercise done three times round, could take up to ten minutes or more, whereas a session of six or eight short-stitch will be two or three minutes. However, in Session Two we recommend building up gradually so that passive concentration remains good quality. You will practise heaviness in the arms only for the first three days of the week. In the latter four days of the week, you will add heaviness in the legs.

Sometimes Autogenic Therapy is taught in an eight-week course, rather than nine. In this case, Sessions One and Two would be combined.

THE THIRD SESSION
INTRODUCTION OF HEAVINESS PART TWO
BEGINNING THE INTENTIONAL EXERCISES

FEEDBACK ON THE WEEK
Following the usual go-round, report back and diary-reading, any issues arising will be dealt with through discussion or demonstration if necessary.

Some group members will have 'gone for it' — practised the recommended amounts, be having vivid dreams, be experiencing lots of autogenic discharge release, and will be immersed in their exercises to the point of accessing old childhood memories. Stories like these are always interesting and encouraging to the rest of the group, but take care not to compare yourself unfavourably with others. Each individual will progress at their own pace.

INTRODUCTION OF THE NEW EXERCISE
- A trigger formula, using one repetition of the dominant arm heavy, to facilitate quick access to the AT state
- Heaviness in all the limbs at once
- Heaviness in the neck and shoulders
- The Peace Formula as an affirmation before closure.

Rationale and Theory of Heaviness in the Neck and Shoulders
Tension is very often carried and stored in the trapezius muscles. These cover the back of the neck, the shoulders and the upper back, forming a diamond shape. This tension can lead to headaches, pain and stiffness in the neck, sometimes dizziness and pain running down the arms. When muscles at the back of the neck contract, pain sensors in the scalp are stretched, which brings knots of tension to the area. For many people, it is a sign of stress.

Emotions are often linked to muscular tension, and in this case we might think of anger or irritation with phrases like: 'He is a pain in the neck'; 'He gets my back up'.

It must be a universal experience to have neck and shoulder pain. There is much common language to endorse it:

- 'He carries the whole world on his shoulders.'
- 'Her shoulders are bowed with her burdens.'
- 'A weight off my shoulders.'

Extending the idea of heaviness to the neck and shoulder area (as seen in Figure 4) is a natural progression in AT — especially given these common experiences.

HEAVINESS IN THE NECK AND SHOULDERS AS A PARTIAL EXERCISE (1)
This formula can be used at any time, with the eyes open when *not* in an autogenic state. It is repeated several times silently, with the mental focus on the area. It reminds the system to stay calm

throughout the day. This needs frequent practice in order to become effective. You may be given small blue dots to use as a reminder. Stick them in places where they will catch the eye, such as on your telephone, watch, diary or computer, or in the car for use when you are stationary. This partial exercise is excellent when used in stressful situations.

Unfortunately, blue dots do not stick well on people, so you can't stick one on your boss's forehead — but you can imagine one!

Initially the response is a local one: dropping of the shoulders. With practice, a more generalised response is experienced — often stopping the stress response in its tracks.

Figure 4: The Neck and Shoulders

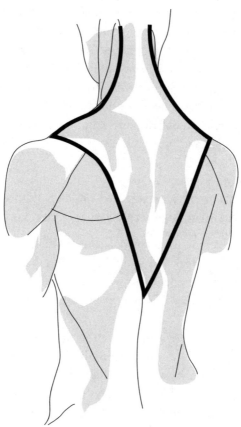

THE PEACE FORMULA

This formula is an affirmation, and is used at the end of an exercise. As it is not linked to a specific part of the body, it gives a summing-up of the exercise experience. It offers a moment when time can be taken to enjoy the effects of the exercise and just be, in a completely passive state, for a short time. At first, there may not be a great feeling of peace — you may even notice some inner conflict — but, with practice, it will come. Sometimes, at the beginning, it may represent an aspiration rather than an affirmation. Or it may be an acceptance that you can be at peace 'at this moment', even with all the aggravation in your life.

INTENTIONAL OFF-LOADING EXERCISES

Throughout the AT course, discussion, explanation and demonstration about how we handle our emotions will be brought into the training. These are dealt with in Chapter 5. Signs of emerging emotional material may be evident at this stage of the autogenic process, and your therapist will probably introduce the early Intentional Exercises. These are the Motor Garbage exercise to off-load physical (muscular) tension, and the Noise Garbage exercise for the voice and breathing.

THE FOURTH SESSION
INTRODUCTION OF WARMTH (STANDARD EXERCISE 2)
BEGIN/CONTINUE THE INTENTIONAL EXERCISES

The whole exercise is adapted again, to include the previous week's formulae (Neck and Shoulders, Peace Formula) and to add in the new formulae relating to warmth in the limbs. This is introduced in the same way as heaviness, by first focusing on each limb in turn.

This week's exercise is the longest in the whole course, but be reassured — it will shorten again the following week. Some people have a 'love–hate' relationship with this exercise — they love it because it is so long, and they hate it because it is so long! We would suggest simply getting the exercises done, and even speeding up the formula repetitions in order to prevent concentration problems. The practice week can again be split into two, focusing first on the arms and then adding the legs in the last few days.

WARMTH: RATIONALE AND THEORY

Observations of people in a deeply relaxed state show that there is a common experience of warmth. As the system responds to the use of heaviness, so feelings of warmth can be experienced quite early on. This may already be indicated by reports of tingling, warmth or sometimes the sense of a pulse somewhere. This may be taken as a demonstration of a reversal of the stress response, where blood which has been diverted, ready for fight and flight, is now free to flow back to the peripheral vessels. We know that when muscles relax, so too do the major and minor blood vessels of the body. This increases blood flow, improving the whole circulatory system, and giving an actual, though minimal, rise in skin temperature.

Heaviness and warmth seem to go in tandem. These two exercises are the foundation of the whole autogenic structure. Schultz and Luthe found that 50 per cent of all improvements in symptoms occurred following the introduction of the two warmth exercises (another one follows in Session Seven).

Sensations of warmth and/or heaviness may be lacking in clients who have had a stroke, head injury or polio, or where the peripheral blood vessels are damaged.

It is helpful, when using the warmth exercise in the early days, not to have the surrounding temperature too extreme, as you could feel uncomfortably hot or cold. This should not be a problem, after using the Warmth exercise for a while.

The exercise is practised in class as before.

THE FIFTH SESSION
INTRODUCTION OF CARDIAC REGULATION EXERCISE
(STANDARD EXERCISE 3)
BEGIN/CONTINUE THE INTENTIONAL EXERCISES

The warmth formulae are shortened to sit alongside the heaviness one, in a combining phrase about heaviness and warmth being present in all the limbs together. There is about four weeks' work in this one phrase, so for this week you will be recommended to increase the repetitions from three, to six or eight. This allows the system to 'take in' the message.

The new formula, relating to the heartbeat being calm and regular, is introduced. This has the potential to increase relaxation and deepens the autogenic state, speeding up the re-balancing process.

The introduction of Intentional Exercises continues.

RATIONALE AND THEORY OF THE HEARTBEAT EXERCISE
It is often observed that during practice of heaviness and warmth in the limbs, the relaxation response has naturally progressed to an awareness of a calming sensation of the heart beating. It is quite common for people to report the feelings of the next exercise before it is introduced: a new formula is only the next stage in a natural process. We never chase a new idea in AT — a formula is simply a confirmation that we are allowing the system to look after itself, as we develop a new self-awareness.

This is the first time that the autogenic programme has 'touched' a major organ, so, as always, we are careful to monitor the process. At this point, before practising the exercise, there may be some discussion in the group about the heart, what it does and what it means to an individual. You may be recommended to place a hand on your chest, so that your awareness is drawn to the area. As you practise, you may be aware of a pulse anywhere in the body. This is fine — self-regulation is already under way.

Sometimes the pulse or heartbeat is quite elusive. If you don't feel it or if it seems to disappear, we would like to be the first to reassure you that your heart has *not* stopped beating! It is only your perception of it that can alter. Focusing on this area for the first time might cause a little anticipatory frisson of anxiety. The feeling during the exercise is that your heartbeat/pulse seems to be racing. All you have to do is observe in the usual casual way, and when you finish the exercise, write your notes.

The key to the cardiac exercise is in allowing the heart to regulate itself. This is usually comforting: you are handing over care of your heartbeat to your own self-righting mechanism. It is looking after you — all you have to do is let it.

If the exercise really feels uncomfortable you can always close (cancel) it before you reach the end. Your therapist will advise about how to modify the formula if you need to. However, nine times out of ten, the 'iffy' effect will occur only on that very first occasion — after that, your brain and body know what to expect, and continue to get on with the job.

Never alter the wording of a formula without your therapist's advice. If you are unhappy about any formula, you can always temporarily leave it out.

THE SIXTH SESSION
INTRODUCTION OF RESPIRATION FORMULA (STANDARD
EXERCISE 4)
CONTINUING THE INTENTIONAL EXERCISES

At this stage, you may well be feeling that you are noticing 'results' in your life: health, attitude, behaviour, response to others, etc. The group will have found its own 'dynamic' — and members will encourage each other.

Your diary may have changed its pattern too. Often it spontaneously changes from a meticulous recording of each and every exercise, to a more general approach. You may be finding that the physiological response to the exercises is pretty much the same each time, and it is the benefits and/or insights outside your practice (the psychological responses) which seem noteworthy — that's fine.

You may also be finding that your practice of Intentional Exercises has a direct relationship with the quality of your AT.

RATIONALE AND THEORY OF BREATHING EXERCISE

In a deep state of relaxation, it is quite natural for the breathing mechanism to slow down. Respiration becomes shallow (sometimes to the point of being imperceptible). In a state of arousal, breathing is deeper; when we are undergoing exercise and effort, the breathing is even more effortful (panting). Here, the heart-rate increases, as does the intake of oxygen, in order for the muscles to work more efficiently.

The breathing mechanism is an involuntary one — we do not have to make a conscious effort to keep breathing. If we did, we would never be able to sleep. However, we do have voluntary control over it. We can breathe in different ways according to different needs — for example, talking, singing, running. Many tasks require us to learn certain breathing techniques, and it is interesting to reflect that this applies to many relaxation techniques as well. Often the first lesson in relaxation techniques is to learn how to 'breathe properly'.

You will now have completed five or six weeks of your AT course, and breathing will not yet have been mentioned in any official way. If the subject has been raised, it will be because of changes in awareness of breathing, or perhaps some awkwardness with it. As long as you remain passive and non-striving, your breathing is fine.

The aim of this formula is to allow the body, without interference from the mind, to let go of conscious control of the breathing function. Practice of the previous AT exercises will already have encouraged a calming and slowing of respiration. Now we introduce a passive awareness of breathing, which is likely to deepen the autogenic state. Often people become aware that they are 'breathing deeper' (tummy breathing) in the exercise. Perhaps the breathing spontaneously comes from the abdomen rather than the upper part of the chest, often becoming slower and shallower.

The formula is quite short, simply bringing attention to your breathing. You will be encouraged to leave a space between each repetition in which to observe. *The task is to let it be.* You might find that you want to take deep breaths, or give big sighs out — that's fine — simply observe that process and go along with it. Your body is breathing for you. You 'follow' the response, you don't lead (control) it.

EXERCISE PATTERN

At this point in the course, your therapist will encourage you to change the style of your exercise pattern. You have now been using AT for a significant period, and as long as your process is stable, you can practise the three exercises without closing (cancelling) in between them. This means that you will be able to maintain the autogenic state of passive awareness for increasing amounts of time, and deepen the autogenic state. It feels pleasurable and very relaxing to abandon the closing in-between.

Sometimes it is not possible to sustain this at first. You might prefer to close the first exercise, and then practise the next two without closing in-between. When this is comfortable, you can do all three in one continuous cycle. You will, of course, always remember to close vigorously at the end.

THE SEVENTH SESSION
INTRODUCTION OF ABDOMINAL WARMTH (STANDARD EXERCISE 5)
CONTINUING THE INTENTIONAL EXERCISES

This session will comprise the usual format and may include discussion of issues around sleep and the Dream Formula (see Chapter 9).

RATIONALE AND THEORY OF ABDOMINAL WARMTH EXERCISE
Reversal of the stress response allows circulation to regulate itself in the abdominal region, usually by increasing blood flow. This produces a warming of the area. As the body is able to enter a deeply relaxed state at will, so abdominal warmth is noticed, espe-

cially as the natural breathing becomes associated with 'coming from a deeper place'.

The formula for warmth in this area is used to enhance the general relaxation response, often resulting in a calming effect. It is frequently linked to an experience of comfort, such as when we cuddle a hot water bottle. As the nervous system becomes increasingly calm, there is often a feeling of drowsiness when muscular tension decreases still further.

The new formula connects us with the solar plexus and completes the overall picture of warmth in autogenic exercises by focusing on the upper abdomen, where emotional tension may be held. The word 'plexus' means 'network of nerves or vessels in an animal body' (*Oxford English Dictionary*). The solar plexus (or gastric plexus) is the meeting point of all the nerve pathways in the body, connecting the brain with the limbs, organs, endocrine and immune systems, etc. The importance of the solar plexus is reflected in its protected position — tucked high in the abdominal cavity, beneath the diaphragm, just in front of the spinal vertebrae, and behind the upper abdominal organs.

We often hear language which reflects its power:

- 'I've got a gut feeling.' (intuition, instinct)
- 'I've got a knot/clenched fist in my stomach.' (anxiety, anger, jealousy)

To enable you to practise this formula in a wider context than 'trying to find that dot in my tummy', your therapist may well suggest another connection — with the philosophy of eastern meditation methods, where the centre of the body is acknowledged as the true centre of the person. This may be interpreted as the 'soul', the 'core of the being', the 'authentic being', the 'true self'.

It doesn't matter whether or not you perceive any warmth in this area. It is enough, in your state of passive awareness, just to keep using the phrase.

This formula is likely to deepen the autogenic state and increase the levels of relaxation.

The practice of Intentional Exercises two or three times a week should be continuing.

THE EIGHTH SESSION
INTRODUCTION OF COOLNESS TO FOREHEAD
(STANDARD EXERCISE 6)
CONTINUING THE INTENTIONAL EXERCISES

Now you are reaching the final stages of the course, and the sixth Standard Exercise completes all the steps of learning AT. As with all the exercises, the idea of the cool forehead evolved from experiences during previous exercises. For example, some people report feeling a slight 'draught' effect on the forehead even while using Heaviness and Warmth in the limbs. This indicates that the relaxation response does not confine itself simply to the exercise we happen to be on. It will occur as soon as we are relaxed, and the different exercises point up each manifestation of relaxation

RATIONALE AND THEORY OF FOREHEAD COOL

Cooling the forehead alongside warming the body has been proven to exert a calming effect on the system. In old-fashioned asylums, treatment of mentally agitated patients used warm baths and cool flannels on the forehead. We have common language to match:

- 'Cool it — calm down'
- 'Cool headed'
- 'I need to chill out.'
- 'Cool as a cucumber'.

Conversely, increased blood supply to the cranial region (your skull, head and brain), with the use of either warmth or heaviness, would be undesirable in an area where the blood supply is already well regulated. Doing this could cause headaches. (We consider being 'hot-headed' or 'heavy-headed' negative attributes.)

Body language often reflects the calming influence of the idea of coolness in the forehead, as when we see people placing a hand on the forehead, or smoothing a fevered brow.

When this sixth and final formula is introduced, you will be encouraged to focus on the forehead or brow, and repeat the new phrase relating to coolness there.

FOREHEAD COOL AS A PARTIAL EXERCISE (2)

This formula can be used as a second partial exercise to encourage a cool, clear head at any time or in any place. Once again, it is silently repeated with eyes open, not in an autogenic state. Its effectiveness will depend on the amount of practice you give it. As a reminder, replace your blue spots with another colour for a week or so, and practise up to 100 times throughout a day.

You have now built up over the weeks the complete set of autogenic formulae which form the final exercise. This is what you will continue to practise.

THE AUTOGENIC PROCESS

If you have experienced a 'bumpy ride' during your process, you will probably find that things are beginning to settle down as all the autogenic formulae are assimilated. From now on, continuing a good level of practice of Standard Exercises and Intentional Exercises is essential, to allow the autogenic process to reach its full potential.

THE NINTH SESSION
INTRODUCTION OF PERSONAL AND MOTIVATIONAL FORMULAE
PERSONAL ASSESSMENT OF THE WHOLE COURSE

This session will include:
The Second Part of Written Self-Reflection
Blood Pressure Checks if Required
The Usual Session Go-round — *reviewing the whole course as well as the previous week*

Introduction of Personal and Motivational Formulae

This will be either Week 8 or Week 9, depending on the format of your course. All the Standard Exercises have been introduced, with all the Intentional Exercises.

The go-round in the final session will focus on all aspects of the group's progress through the course, as well as their experience of the last exercise (SE6).

WRITTEN SELF-REFLECTION — SECOND PART

(This second part of the exercise is sometimes left until the follow-up session.)

On a clean sheet of paper, you will reflect on, and write about, the AT course as a whole. This will take about ten minutes. It is useful to think about what is going on in your life, now that you are in the habit of using AT. You wrote down a self-portrait at the start of the course — 'Me in My Life Now' — on life at home and at work, health, relationships, hobbies, fun, etc. Do it again now.

When you have finished writing, you will read your first sheet. It is up to you if you want to share your thoughts about it, or parts of them. If you are doing an individual course, this can be a good time to go through things in more detail with your therapist.

You may be encouraged to try this written exercise again later on — say in six months' time — in which case you will then have a third sheet to compare with these two. It can be seen as an ongoing life-assessment check.

You may well be surprised at some of the differences. Examples of common responses are:

- 'I'd forgotten all the headaches I was getting then — I haven't had one for weeks.'
- 'Oh — wasn't I in state then?'

REVIEW OF THE COURSE

The go-round will include brief discussion of the two sheets. You will be encouraged to seek out any differences in the style of writing each sheet, as well as focusing on content. There is often surprise that change has happened without your being consciously aware of it. For example, a few short bullet points may have changed to flowing prose; certain words, such as 'worry' may not have appeared at all on the second sheet, whereas they were prominent in the first.

INTRODUCTION OF PERSONAL AND MOTIVATIONAL FORMULAE
See Chapter 6.

PREPARE FOR THE FOLLOW-UP
You will be reassured that the group will be meeting again in four, six or eight weeks' time. This is an important stage to come, and gives a chance to review progress and check things out.

ON-GOING THERAPIST CONTACT
Your therapist will always encourage you to make contact if any problems should arise. Maybe an individual chat is necessary if you feel that you are left with unresolved issues, and uncertainties as to how to deal with them. Do you need further help? Even if you feel that the answer to that question is 'yes', it is always a good idea to leave it for a while, let the autogenic process work a little more, and see how things settle down. Some people need to reach the end of the course and get on with their lives without feeling that they have to come to a class each week and tell people how they are doing. Finishing the course can raise some issues about endings, letting go, moving on. Let these happen, use your Intentional Exercises, and reassess in a few weeks.

THE TENTH SESSION
THE FOLLOW-UP

This is usually arranged for six to eight weeks after the last AT session. Your therapist may have sent you a reminder letter, possibly with a post-course questionnaire, in order to help you to assess your progress. Learning AT with regular weekly support from a trained therapist is a different thing from being 'out in the world' on your own with it.

Elements of the follow-up session are discussed more fully in Chapter 4.

FOLLOW-UP SESSION STRUCTURE

- Practice of Full AT Standard Exercise — Revision
- Go-round/Feedback on the Previous Few Weeks
  - How effective is/was your Personal Formula?
  - Do you need to change/add to it?
- Reminders about Intentional (off-loading) Exercises
- Completion of any Post-Course Assessment Questionnaires Your Therapist Recommends
- Final Group Exercises:
  - Standard Exercise (perhaps with the option of using a wordless form)
  - Space Exercise
- How to Use AT in the Future
- How to Extend Your Exercises
- How to Get Going Again After a Break in AT Practice
- Building on to Your New-Found Skills
- Keeping Linked to AT through Each Other? (or being Friend of the BAS)

CHAPTER 4

MORE ABOUT THE COURSE

THE GROUP SETTING

Essentially the autogenic group is a class, where several people have come together to learn AT for a variety of reasons. The aim is the same for everyone; the individual reasons for being there are not divulged unless you wish (unlike group psychotherapy). What you do share are your AT experiences.

It is important to agree ground rules in the group. You will be asked to observe group discipline, which involves punctuality, letting the therapist know if you have to arrive late, or have to miss the session. We respect confidentiality in the group. 'If you hear it here, leave it here.'

Also, you will be advised to keep AT to yourself. Just as you should not be learning from anyone but a qualified therapist, neither should you attempt to teach anyone else. Simple as AT seems, and enthusiastic as you may be, it is not wise to go home after the session and show your interested relatives what you have been doing: everyone responds differently. Even if you talk about it, you may find others sceptical as they do not understand what AT is — this can undermine your motivation. It's your business, not theirs — just keep the details to yourself.

THE MISSED GROUP SESSION

Every therapist will have their own ways of making sure you do not miss out if you unavoidably have to miss a session. Depending on factors such as geography or time, you may be offered a short catch-up session (for which a charge may be made), or you might catch up by telephone, e-mail or post. In any event, the responsibility of catching up lies with you, the client.

The Training Diary

At first, your response to autogenic exercises is often very subtle, and practice is needed to raise awareness of the fleeting effects. We are usually too busy to notice the messages our bodies give us, or we ignore them. To understand these subtle signals, we first need to learn how to observe them, so your therapist will recommend that you keep a written record throughout your course.

You may be supplied with a small notebook for the purpose, to keep with you, and private, at all times. Each time you do an exercise, after the final close and reflection, you will make brief notes on what you observed. This may seem something of an unnecessary chore at first, but don't give up. Any observation, written down, is an acknowledgement of your process, even if it seems trivial and irrelevant.

You are paying attention to yourself, and keeping the diary actively helps your autogenic process. The diary will reflect your early stages of effort, where you are 'just doing it' — applying the instructions and generally getting the hang of it. You will need to bring it to each weekly session, and your therapist will read it, but they will never disclose anything personal in it. However, occasionally a technical point might be picked up, if the therapist regards it as useful for the group as a whole. Your therapist will be looking for signs that you are encouraging passive concentration by setting up the best possible environment when you can.

The authors have both felt frustrated time and again in a group session, when the diary of a member looks like this:

Monday 5th		*Tuesday 6th*	
8.00 a.m.	✓	*7.30 a.m.*	✓
Lunchtime	✓	*Lunchtime*	✓
8.30 p.m.	✓	*7.45 p.m.*	✓

and then, when they tell us about their week, all kinds of things have been going on. For example, they have been getting back pain in every exercise; dreaming vividly and in glorious technicolor;

feeling not so rushed during the day; scratchy and irritable with the family; caught up in childhood memories.

'So why is none of this in the diary?' we ask.

'I didn't think it was important,' is the usual reply.

Everything is important in AT. In time, you will not be judging — you will be accepting all your experiences as relevant. There is no right or wrong response.

If you know that you are going to have to write something in your diary, and you know that your therapist will read it each week, you will pay proper attention to each exercise.

If you do not like writing, let us reassure you that the diary can be very brief: just a line or two for each exercise — no complete sentences necessary, and there will definitely be no spelling corrections! You might choose to use your computer if that feels easier.

After each exercise the following information should be recorded:

- The week number with day or date
- The time of day of exercise
- The duration of the exercise — measure and record this once or twice during a week
- The posture used
- The type of exercise (short-stitch, standard, etc.)
- The formulae used (if different from the recommended ones for the week)
- Any phone contact you have had with your therapist and a record of their suggestions.
- Frequent experiences during the exercise — *e.g. 'slight headache starting in second exercise', 'ache in left chest', 'pain in big toe', 'lots of intruding thoughts', 'felt like crying', 'felt restless & had to stop', 'did not want to close', 'saw a black hole', 'felt apprehensive', etc.*
- Effects of the exercise — *e.g. relaxed, comfortable, tingling, tummy rumbles, better mood after, less tense after, few distractions, etc.*
- New training symptoms — *e.g. heaviness in both legs, warmth in the arms.*

- Occasional experiences (discharges) — *e.g. 'feel like spinning', 'electricity down my arm', 'saw an eye looking at me', 'felt like sliding', 'felt lop-sided', 'arm seemed very long', 'pulsating', etc.*
- Difficulties — such as posture, interruptions, time, environment, etc.
- A record of partial exercises practised
- A record of which Intentional Off-loading Exercises and when; how long they lasted; your experiences during them; any difficulties; any effect they had on subsequent Standard Exercises.
- Any queries.
- Daily summary: we suggest that you write any general comments at the end of a day — *e.g. sleep patterns, dreams, mood changes, etc.*

Your diary gives to your therapist a wealth of information, which is entirely individual: clues as to your ability to use passive concentration; timings of exercises affecting their outcomes; whether you are going too fast or too slow; whether you are doing too few or too many repeats; whether your discharge activity is becoming uncomfortable; whether you are neglecting any of the postures. Coupled with verbal feedback, your diary helps the therapist to monitor your progress, which will help you to feel able to proceed with confidence.

You may love writing, and be only too happy to fill screeds of paper each week. This is probably less of a diary and more of a journal, and there's no harm in that. Your journal entries will help you to discover more insights about yourself. However, if you wish to use this style, we recommend that you keep two diaries: one for the journal, the other your brief notes for the AT session, as this is easier for the therapist to manage in the group setting.

Whatever your chosen style, do make sure that your diary is absolutely private.

DO I HAVE TO CONTINUE KEEPING MY DIARY WHEN THE COURSE HAS FINISHED?

You will be encouraged to keep something going, at least up to the follow-up session. Perhaps you will do a weekly summary, or a record of anything significant — be it insight or new AT experience. If you found the discipline of keeping the diary a useful one, you might choose to continue it in the form of a journal. This can be used to explore feelings, life-changes, etc. However you choose to do it, keeping up the diary does help motivation.

THE AUTOGENIC DISCHARGE

Modern research says that the mind and body hold on to the memory of all experience, and that most of this memory is beyond our conscious control. Regression methods can trigger and raise these memories, and so can any relaxation or meditation method. Autogenic Therapy is no different in this respect, and Schultz gave a name to this phenomenon: the autogenic discharge.

Unexpressed emotions are often held in muscles. Wilhelm Reich described body 'armouring' as a way in which we un-consciously choose to protect ourselves from uncomfortable emotions. As years go by, with these tensions left unresolved, the emotional memories are buried while the physical pain increases. If you consider how your muscles react when you hold in anger or stop yourself from crying, you will become aware of tension in many of them. When you are in a state of anxiety, look at where your shoulders are held, and note the tension in your neck.

The body's memories of physical or emotional trauma are intact. As the autogenic process deepens, the body and mind are given a golden opportunity to off-load some of these accumulated tensions quite spontaneously as part of the healthy self-regulation process. Unless these are disturbingly uncomfortable, they should be passively accepted.

These discharges are normally at a very low intensity and are merely observed in a passive state as mild sensations or tics or twitches. They may be easily explained as relating to a past physical trauma, such as a tooth extraction, or a cut finger.

Example

> 'In one of my exercises I had a pain in my mouth which reminded me of when I had a tooth out as a child. I then felt pressure on my face, which felt like a mask, and had to stop the exercise because I couldn't breathe.'

There was no repeat of this experience in subsequent exercises. The brain had done its job. This person needed calm reassurance that the off-loading of that dental experience was quite normal, and that her body had healed itself of that past traumatic experience.

Example

> 'Twenty years ago I know I sliced the end off my finger at work. I didn't remember which finger it was until my AT exercise, and I got a sharp pain which felt like that accident. I needed to "nurse" it for a few moments — it never happened again.'

This man was astonished at the vivid feelings of his healing process, and fascinated by the depth at which AT can work. It encouraged him to witness his process in this way, and, far from being afraid, he found that his interest in AT increased.

Some discharges may be directly linked to an unresolved emotion, such as grief. This might emerge in the form of watering eyes or twitching eyelids, tension across the nose or a lump in the throat. Sometimes discharges are in a visual form ('in the mind's eye') and may be of faces, eyes, or objects.

Other discharges may be sensations of bodily movement or distortion, such as in the following examples: *'I felt that the right side of my body was much smaller than the left.' 'I felt as though I was sitting on my own lap.' 'I felt as though I was leaning right over to one side, although I knew I wasn't.' 'I felt curled up in a nice warm place.'* These are manifestations of self-righting adjustments taking place.

Discharges may emerge in the form of feelings, such as joy and love. Or memories evocative of childhood can hold our attention perhaps for a few hours or a day. Apprehension, anger or sadness can similarly move us, both during exercises and after them.

Memories involving all the senses may arise. Smells, or perceptions of touch, along with tastes, sounds and images are all possible when in an altered state of consciousness, as shown in the following examples:

- *I had a strong memory of the smell of pine forests in New Zealand — it was a vivid reminder of home.*
- *Suddenly, in the second cycle of the exercise, I smelt my mother's perfume. It felt as though she were standing beside me, but she lives 100 miles away.*
- *I thought the chair I was sitting on had had new covers — I could feel silky velvet under my fingers.*
- *I felt I was submerged in water, it seemed to cling to the whole body, but I could still breathe — no distress at all.*
- *I heard faint music for a few seconds.*
- *I'm sure I heard the engine of a Rolls Royce — it didn't seem to fade — just stayed where it was until I closed.*
- *I saw the house I lived in when I was seven.*
- *In the third cycle there was a face — I didn't know who it was. It disappeared before I finished the exercise.*
- *I saw a stick — just hanging in my field of vision. I closed the exercise as I felt a bit uneasy.*

In the rare event that images should begin to move, like 'film strips' in the mind, you would be advised to close. They may herald unpleasant feelings and are usually associated with some memory of mind-disturbing material, such as bad trips on drugs, delirium, or severe head injury. There is nothing wrong with this process, as your mind is always working towards rebalance. But we encourage you to stay within the structure of the exercise, rather than engaging with the potentially disturbing dream-like state.

Interpretation of such material is not essential. We simply understand the process to be beneficial. However, it can be useful to note the variety of the discharge, as this can be linked to a particular emotional build-up, and may therefore be a guide to the required Intentional Off-loading Exercise (see Chapter 5).

Occasionally, discharges will be quite distracting. These can be managed by reducing the focus of the autogenic formula or shortening the Standard Exercise. Intentional Off-loading Exercises will help to discharge the emotional backlog and relieve the symptoms, and then normal Standard Exercises can be resumed.

WHAT IF I DON'T GET ANY DISCHARGES?

Not everyone experiences noticeable discharges, and you should not feel that their absence is any indication that things are not going well. There will be other signs that your therapist will look for to confirm your progress.

INTRUDING THOUGHTS

In the early stages of practising AT, clients are often anxious that they are not practising adequately, and they can try too hard to banish intrusion, almost as if punishing themselves. Everyone has patches of practice where they are seemingly thinking of anything and everything except the exercise.

Bear in mind that our westernised culture is not conducive to emptying the mind — we are not in the habit of meditating for long periods, and all the grey matter of the brain is still functioning even though we are doing AT. If we try to empty or 'blank' the mind, we will fail. So, it is best to accept what is there and take a mild interest in it, while continuing with the exercise. A 70:30 ratio in passive concentration is generally considered acceptable: 70 per cent of your attention on the exercise; 30 per cent on other thoughts.

How to Manage Intruding Thoughts

In the early days of a course, some awareness is needed to deal with the amount of intrusion, in order to develop the ability to use passive concentration. We need to learn what the 'autogenic state' feels like, and how to stay there for a time without disintegration of it.

There are two varieties of intruding thought, and these are described as follows:

1: Intruding Thoughts Related to Current Events

It is common to think about your life, your work, and how to do an AT exercise. These thoughts can be reduced by preparing the ground for your AT.

- Clear the mind of tasks: write them down so you don't have to remember them.
- Time your AT between other activities of the day: before starting the day, after leaving home, before starting work, after work, before evening activities.

Other possible ways of dealing with such thoughts would be:
- Speed up the formula repetitions, leaving less time for thoughts to intrude
- Change the environment (go to a quiet bedroom instead of a noisy family room)
- Practise short-stitch before beginning. This will help to quieten the 'mind-chatter'.

2. Intruding Thoughts Related to the Autogenic Process

As the course progresses and the autogenic state deepens, the character of intruding thoughts may change, with the thoughts tending to be random memories, random thoughts, creative ideas, thoughts unrelated to current day-to-day activity. In this situation, the usual attitude of passive acceptance is maintained, and formula repetition is continued.

Strong emotional thought which continually pulls you away from the autogenic formula repetition may cause passive concentration to be lost, and the exercise should be ended. This might indicate the need to use Intentional Off-loading Exercises. Sometimes it is necessary to sacrifice an Autogenic session for an Intentional one. The result will be a clearing out of emerging emotional content, and the next autogenic exercise *will feel easier to practise, with fewer distractions.*

RESISTANCE

Autogenic exercises are easy to learn: they are based on mental repetition of simple phrases, carried out in particular conditions. We all know that we can learn almost anything if we are prepared to apply ourselves diligently, to do as we are instructed and to practise enough. And yet, in some cases, we simply don't do it. Why not? Something within us resists change — perhaps it is fear of the unknown, moving into a different way of being, or into unfamiliar territory where our behaviour has to change — suddenly we are confronted by our own internal saboteurs.

When you have become used to being in a permanent state of tension, you may feel a little insecure as you begin to let go in your exercises. You imagine that there is a fault with the technique — your motivation to practise could slip even further. Or you are afraid of 'getting it wrong' or 'showing yourself up': *'I can't do it properly.' 'It's not for me.'*

Learning AT means taking time for yourself, but we are not used to taking care of our own needs and often feel guilty about practising. Our education teaches us never to waste time, that sitting for ten minutes doing nothing is wrong — so, when your eyes are closed in a state of passive concentration, this can seem unproductive and selfish.

When new habits are not firmly fixed, it is all too easy to revert to the familiar old ways, even if these are unhealthy or destructive. So you may find yourself avoiding practice — you will 'just finish this' before you do your exercises. All sorts of displacement activities creep in: cleaning out cupboards, washing the car, or doing a whole range of urgent things that you have already put off for years. You may find yourself cutting corners — rushing through the exercise, using an incorrect posture, trying it while watching your favourite TV programme, inviting interruption by not telling others you are going to practise. Or you might do the exercises without first making sure that you have a good environment, or checking out the new formula.

We have heard all the excuses before, and we recognise them as resistance. '*I was out so I couldn't practise.*' '*We had visitors.*' '*My cat got sick.*' You won't fool your therapist, so once you begin to hear your own excuses and understand that your internal saboteur is working against you, you can find solutions to these difficulties.

For example, using AT at work will be invaluable for you in the future. Try getting into the habit of taking a break at lunchtime and, if possible, leaving the building — it helps the rest of the day to be much more effective. Or you can do a quick exercise with your back to the rest of the room, and using a discreet close. Some people find ingenious ways of fitting in their AT right from the start, despite open-plan offices and no coffee- or lunch-break. If you resist doing your exercises at work, you may never get the habit.

Tell people what you're doing — ask for a little space, rather than struggle on, getting more and more frustrated by being continually interrupted.

Be fussy about setting up good conditions in the early weeks of practice, and you will be setting yourself up to tolerate less than perfect conditions in the future. Some practice in adverse conditions is inevitable (using time on the train is excellent, if sometimes a bit fraught).

In addition, as you begin to make new and subtle changes in your attitude and behaviour, those close to you may also find that they have to adapt. Here, *they* may have the resistance to *your* change.

When you return from the first week's practice, having completed a reasonable number of exercises in the recommended conditions, you will know that you are making progress. However, if frustrations and resistances have crept in, it is easy to perceive yourself as 'a failure'. It may be difficult to 'get going', and even turning up to the second session is hard. By the end, after reassuring discussion where others will have said similar things, you will be relieved and encouraged, and glad that you came.

If the first week's practice is lost, it is not the end of the world. As you face up to the responsibility that AT won't do itself, you will resolve to pick up the exercises from that point and go on to do really well. This is the advantage of having only short-stitch to practise in the early days. If the full heaviness exercise (Session Two) is introduced at the start, and resistance prevents practice, a very important week's work will have been missed.

Sometimes resistance to practice can be a protection against uncomfortable material emerging too quickly. Your therapist will help you to recognise this, the autogenic programme will be adapted, and Intentional Off-loading Exercises will be used.

SHORT-STITCH AS AUTOGENIC 'FIRST AID'

The short-stitch exercise was developed to allow a very brief visit to the autogenic state. It uses repetition of the trigger phrase, interspersed with frequent closure (cancelling). When these short exercises are strung together, they give a calming effect without great demand upon passive concentration. A training posture should be used, and a brief scan at the start. There may be no apparent effect at first, but the autogenic process is triggered, and the effects will follow.

If a longer exercise is too difficult to sustain for any reason, we would recommend that you revert to short-stitch for a day or a few days. This will keep the autogenic process going, while reducing its intensity.

Short-stitch is used:

- When passive concentration is poor and a full exercise is not possible
- When there is anger, distress or anxiety — several short-stitch exercises together may exert a calming influence, and then allow a longer exercise to follow

- When there is restricted time — you can take two minutes for yourself
- When in too much pain to focus on a longer exercise
- When someone is feeling ill, and concentration on long exercises is not possible —in such cases, short-stitch can help the mind and body to drift into a healing sleep.

Short-stitch is a very useful exercise throughout life. It can be used to calm the system when agitated or uncomfortable. If three repeats of the formula feel too much, two repeats can be used. Even this brief exercise is very effective.

Maintaining AT Practice

Often, when the course is coming to an end, there are worries and concerns about keeping AT going. It is still early days, and the self-righting process will be continuing. You now have the tools to continue on your own with, perhaps, minimal help from the therapist. By now you will be familiar with how AT fits in with your daily routine, and you may be resolved to keep going with that. The regular 3x3 pattern is always the best option. Your brain is consistently 'plugging into' your self-righting processes — it is now familiar with acting on the autogenic instructions very quickly.

Maybe, after a while, you will have cut your practice down to twice a day: one day-time and one night-time exercise. Maybe you will feel guilty that the night exercise is a 'cheat', because you go to sleep so quickly, and you don't get very far. This is fine — the brain likes to go to sleep in the autogenic state, which wears off spontaneously. Even using the trigger phrase alone will achieve this. We certainly don't want you staying awake in order to complete your autogenic exercise — if your system is ready for sleep, go with it.

The Neutral State

Neutral State — The 'No-Thought Phase'
In the latter stages of your AT course, you may be finding yourself sometimes 'lost' in the autogenic state, in a pleasant, thoughtless

reverie. There are no other thoughts, and after a brief time you suddenly 'come to', knowing that you have let go of the exercise, and you haven't been to sleep yet you feel refreshed. Luthe described this as a 'no-thought phase'.

How Do I Know when I am in the Neutral State?
You might expect that you would never know if you had been in a 'no-thought' state. You will have stopped using autogenic phrases, you will not have been asleep and you will not be thinking about anything else. Often you might 'come to' and think that by losing concentration your exercise has been rendered invalid or a waste of time. Far from it. When we describe this state to our clients, there is usually a nod of recognition when we say, 'but you know you haven't been to sleep'. It seems that the brain can get into such a deep *yet alert* altered state — it can 'coast along in neutral'.

Awareness that this 'other place' has been reached often occurs with the heaviness and warmth formulae or the breathing formula. You will need plenty of practice in order to experience the neutral state, but please do not seek it out — no striving is necessary. As long as the drift away from the formulae does not contain other thoughts or feelings, but remains genuinely empty, you can be assured that you are in the neutral state.

VARIATIONS OF THE STANDARD EXERCISES

THE MAINTENANCE EXERCISES
These may be introduced either in Session Nine or at the follow-up, in order to offer some alternatives to the full 3x3 programme. The first maintenance exercise is constructed in a slightly different format from the 3x3, and is practised as a one-off, not as a cycle of three repeats. The second version is shorter, and uses heaviness and warmth formulae only. Both maintenance exercises are very useful when time is short.

Some people use them only two or three times a week; others stick to their familiar 3x3 regime. The choice is yours, although it is good to bear in mind that more practice is always better than less.

THE STAND-BY EXERCISE

Sometimes known as the 'Hold' exercise, this combines the heaviness and warmth formulae with 'neck and shoulders' and 'peace'. It is used if the course needs to be held up for a week or so, often between Sessions Four and Five of a nine-week course. It is excellent for preparing the brain for the introduction of the cardiac formula (Standard Exercise 3), while consolidating the longer heaviness and warmth exercises.

HOW TO EXTEND YOUR EXERCISES

As you become more proficient at reaching and maintaining the autogenic state, you may like to extend the exercises. This can be done in a number of ways:

- You may use more repeats of each formula, thereby staying longer in each phase of the exercise.
- You may repeat the whole exercise more than three times.
- You could add the Space Exercise on to the end of the Standard Exercise.

The longer that you stay in the autogenic state, the more opportunity you are giving your system to regulate itself.

Caution: If there is still a need to off-load any emotional material, you will find it very difficult to maintain passive concentration for an extended time. In this case, keep the autogenic exercises short, and use the Intentional Off-loading Exercises.

THE FOLLOW-UP SESSION — SHALL I GO?

Reaching the full potential of any of the autogenic formulae can take several weeks or months, so it makes sense to let some time elapse before the follow-up session. It is interesting to observe how some people who may not have practised very much during this time have still continued positive progress.

You may have decided that you won't go because you have dropped practice a bit. However, it is very important that you attend, as you may find new insights or tips about your practice, which will be most helpful for the future. Your therapist will be only too pleased to help you get the most out of the work you have already done.

This session is a good time to check out how you are doing — an opportunity to remind yourself of the methods, discuss your use of AT, Intentional Off-loading Exercises and personal formulae, and to look towards future support and self-development, if required.

SPACE EXERCISES

These two exercises are not part of the standard programme. However they are a very useful adjunct to it, sometimes as a variant on the autogenic theme. The First Space Exercise is often used as an introduction, perhaps as a demonstration at a lecture on AT; here it can stand on its own. It can also be used as a precursor to a Standard Exercise, or the Standard Exercise can be an introduction to the Space Exercise. These uses are only appropriate for more experienced users of AT, as the deep meditative state is prolonged. It should not be used in this way during a period of significant off-loading. So in the right circumstances a Standard Exercise leading into the Space Exercise is a good preparation for using the Autogenic Meditative Exercises (see Chapter 11). The first Space Exercise is also very useful for helping sleep and to help lower high blood pressure.

It is likely that you will be taught this exercise towards the end of the course, or at the follow-up session. The second Space Exercise is used specifically for lowering high blood pressure, in which case regular monitoring needs to be undergone with your therapist.

DOING THE FIRST SPACE EXERCISE
The principle of passive observation is exactly the same as when practising Standard Exercises. The phrases relate to an imagined idea of space, both within and around various parts of the body, starting with the eyes and ears, and ending with the legs and feet.

The only task is to observe and experience the feelings which arise when using the phrases. If anything disturbing occurs, you will use the same closing method as for the Standard Exercises. If you are using it to help sleep, you will not close – simply allow yourself to drift into sleep. Usually people experience a generalised feeling of relaxation, which may well encompass spontaneous heaviness and warmth.

How to Use AT in the Future

The frequency of your AT practice using the Standard Exercises will determine the speed of your progress. If you are aware that there is more work to be done, regular sessions of two or three times per day will keep you moving forward.

Remember: fewer exercises — slower progress.

You may wish just to maintain your present status, so one or two exercises a day will keep you on an even keel. If you feel that things are not going so well *('I feel stressed again; I had a bad headache again — the first for ages')*, you can step up the frequency.

If you feel ill or distressed, passive concentration may be difficult. Don't struggle to do long exercises — remember short-stitch in its various forms. 'Little and often' may suit better.

How to Get Going Again After a Break

It seems that outside circumstances will often get in the way of our best intentions to keep going with AT. Without the regular encouragement of the training sessions, things can slip. In our view, the commonest times for slips are Saturdays, holidays and Christmas.

Don't worry if your practice lapses for a few days, weeks, or even months — all is not lost. You will be able to pick it up again very fast. AT is like riding a bike — once learned, you never lose the basic skill.

You will be more self-aware by now, and will probably notice if you are slipping into old patterns and behaviours, and you will resolve to do something about it. Start again with short-stitch, dip your toe in the water, and discover how delicious it is to meet with your 'old friend' (AT) again. Do little and often, and build up slowly, practising in a good environment, when you are at your most relaxed. If you have not used your Standard Exercise for some time, it will be the ability to use passive concentration that you will need to regain.

Many people will return to their AT at a time of stress. In this case, you probably need to deal first with an accumulation of tension — emotional or physical. Use the Intentional Off-loading Exercises for this, remembering that their purpose is to clear out and cleanse.

REFRESHER SESSIONS
Your therapist will usually offer the opportunity to have refresher sessions to get you back on track if necessary.

Can I Start the Course Again?
You can start at the beginning and build the whole programme, step-by-step, just as you did in your original course. You have all the material, and you will know the basics. There is no need to spend a whole week on each step — a day or two will suffice. Do bear in mind, though, that you could embark on further off-loading by doing this. Starting again can be a bit like seeing a film for the second time — this time you know the story, and you can pay more attention to the detail. You might let your therapist know that you are doing this, so that you can contact them if you encounter difficulties.

AT Without Words
It is sometimes the case that the longer you practise AT, the more routine it can become — even to the extent that repeating phrases over and over can feel like a 'by rote' chore, rather than allowing a true switch into effortless mindful awareness. It is as though the words get in the way.

A natural progression of practice often emerges spontaneously, as clients and therapists alike realise that they can tap into autogenic exercises without using the phrases. This is not for everyone, and not for every circumstance, but it does encourage the mind-focus to connect more intensely with the body.

Doing AT without using the words is effective only when you are really familiar with it, and using it regularly. Then you will trust that your brain needs only a minimal 'nudge' to remind itself of the task. After the usual preliminaries of adopting posture and attitude, use the trigger phrase to start you off. Then, simply take your awareness to your arms and legs. Stay focused there for a few moments. The chances are you will notice heaviness and warmth. However, you may also notice your breathing, a pulse somewhere, and whole-body warmth, with a cool forehead as well. Every few seconds, direct your attention to the 'sites' of the autogenic exercises, and enjoy! You will quickly realise how integrated the whole is: we do not have to wait for an effect — it is already there.

CHAPTER 5

EMOTIONAL IMPLICATIONS OF LEARNING AT: INTENTIONAL OFF-LOADING EXERCISES

*A*n autogenic process has the potential for profound healing on all levels. However, intruding thoughts which relate to discharge activity can make passive concentration difficult. The presence of this material could cause resistance to practising autogenic exercises, especially as the relaxation feels less effective. Over time, and with adaptation of the Standard Exercises, this off-loading might work itself through, but prior to the development of the Intentional Off-loading Exercises, the autogenic course could take many months. A great degree of motivation was required to stick with the learning process and, unsurprisingly, many trainees dropped out.

Something was needed to enhance the process of off-loading, and restore the pleasant experiences and other recuperative benefits of the Standard Autogenic Exercises.

In 1982, Dr Luthe introduced to British therapists the Intentional Off-loading Exercises, and there is no doubt of their value. These exercises are complementary to the autogenic exercises, running alongside them as an extra aid to speeding up and working through the re-balancing process. Over years of clinical observation and research, Luthe identified consistent physical manifestations of suppressed emotional material. This links in with other modern research into the effects upon health of our emotions: suppressed anger and heart disease; anxiety and the speed of recovery from surgery.

WHAT ARE INTENTIONAL EXERCISES?

These exercises carry a specific intent, unlike autogenic exercises. As we shall see, unexpressed emotions can be stored, and they need release, either through working with the body, or through working directly with the emotions. These exercises can be selected for a specific purpose, with the expected outcome of release and a task completed. We would remind you that autogenic exercises carry no such intent of specific outcome. For clarity, we refer to these exercises as Intentional Off-loading Exercises.

The Intentional Off-loading Exercises mimic nature's ways of dealing with emotional triggers. They provide a fast and efficient way of attending to the discharge of such material by copying the innate uninhibited response to life events. When these are used in conjunction with the Standard Exercises, a return to balanced functioning is greatly speeded up, enabling the autogenic process to be completed in a matter of weeks. In the meantime, clients increase their insight and also develop the skills to progress on their own.

Natural expression of emotions has been a problem for humans for many years, especially in western cultures. Social conditioning has taught us to suppress an outward show of emotion. Even today, gender conditioning still influences the suppression of certain emotions. Boys are 'sissy' if they cry — but it is OK for them to be angry; girls must be 'nice' — but aggression is not acceptable. We must all maintain a 'stiff upper lip' in the face of tears or fear.

When we resist an impulse for natural emotional release, the unexpressed emotion (such as a need to cry) is stored and held as tension in the body. This may lead to a range of physical and psychological problems which cause 'dis-ease' and may even lead to disease. Some of these symptoms are described as psychosomatic (see Chapter 7), and may have been 'around' for many years, no longer consciously associated with the original trigger. Examples of these symptoms are frontal headaches, chest pain, and unexplained joint pains where no injury has occurred.

Suppressed emotional material may come from childhood trauma, from major events in life or from a steady exposure to stressful events over time. Although such past events may be considered over and done with, there are usually residues of effect which linger. This stored material can be resurrected in a variety of ways: when similar events recur; when places of trauma are revisited; when meeting with certain people from the past; when similar events appear in the media. These reminders can stir up uncomfortable feelings or mood swings, which may or may not be recognised as linked with the past.

Only when suppressed material has been released are we able to move on and not be affected by these reminders.

During the practice of Standard Autogenic Exercises, as the mind and body work together towards homeostasis (optimum balanced functioning), right-brain activity allows the beneficial release of accumulated emotional material (see Chapter 7). This can start as early as the first introduction to heaviness, although, for many trainees, discharge activity starts as the process deepens after three or four weeks. Much of the time, this off-loading process is barely discernible, but it can become uncomfortable, and disturb the relaxing nature of the Standard Exercises.

With the introduction of each new autogenic formula, focusing on a different part of the body, new emotional discharge might surface. This reflects areas of the body where an individual might have stored emotional material. For example, the breathing formula (SE4) may give rise to suppressed anxiety symptoms; the abdominal warmth formula (SE5) may release symptoms of suppressed anger.

To give the most benefit, Off-loading Exercises need to be used in conjunction with the Standard Exercises. Training symptoms are reported and observations made. These reports enable the therapist to support trainees in learning how to manage their own processes. Some therapists use a special checklist for autogenic reactions to help in this regard. Intentional Exercises may need to be used frequently at first, in order to deal with accumulated material. This process can be quite short-lived. Later, these exercises become occasional tools for use when an event has upset us. This maintains homeostasis by preventing further build-up of unexpressed material.

The Intentional Off-loading Exercises are always carried out in private, and offer lifelong tools for coping with issues as they occur. Regular use builds up a familiarity, both of the exercises and of your own emotional responses. You will be able to prevent further build-up of the physical and psychological repercussions of suppressed emotions.

These exercises can also be used in anticipation of a stressful event. We can find ourselves thinking about what may happen, and stir up emotional feelings of anxiety, aggression or sadness. If these feelings are off-loaded before the event, a completely different outcome may be experienced.

Example

If the prospect of visiting your mother-in-law stirs up hostile feelings because you always find yourself arguing with her, try off-loading the frustration/irritation before you go, and you could be surprised at the difference in the encounter. You may also avoid coming home with the usual headache.

The five main Intentional Exercises address anger (*Intentional Verbalisation of Aggression*), grief and sadness (*Intentional Crying Exercise*); anxiety (*Intentional Verbalisation of Anxiety*); muscular tension and restlessness (*Intentional Motor Garbage Exercise*); vocal cord constriction and tight breathing (*Intentional Noise Garbage Exercise*).

The Intentional Exercises are often introduced in the following order.

1. INTENTIONAL MOTOR GARBAGE EXERCISE — IMGE (PHYSICAL OFF-LOADING EXERCISE)

We can all identify with the problem of carrying tension around in the body. It is often noticed in the neck and shoulders, but any ache or pain can signify a storing-up of tension. Dr Luthe's name for this exercise relates to the muscular system in the body being known as the 'motor system'.

You may choose to do this exercise when you experience:

- Involuntary movements or twitches during AT exercises
- Feelings of restlessness in the limbs
- Extreme muscle tension.

You may choose to do it:

- Before and after physical activity
- Before relaxation and sleep.

During a restless night, you might decide to give up on the tossing and turning, and get out of bed, go where the floorboards don't creak, and carry out this exercise for a few seconds or minutes. When you get back into bed, you will have released the physical tension, and the body will be better prepared to resume the relaxed state of sleep.

The purpose of the IMGE is to off-load accumulated, unused motor-impulse material, stored as muscular tension. Releasing this tension restores the chemical balance of the muscles, which enables easier relaxation. This exercise is often introduced alongside the heaviness exercise, when focus on the limbs can encourage motor discharges in the form of restless limbs, twitching, or mild aches and pains.

After a moment of standing quietly, eyes closed, and becoming aware of body tension, the eyes are opened, and the limbs are very loosely shaken in uncoordinated movements. Legs, arms, trunk, neck and shoulders are all involved. A series of these movements will last from ten to thirty seconds. To end the exercise, a normal 'close' might be used, but this is not compulsory.

You may well 'feel the wobble'! It is similar to how a dog shakes off the water after swimming. This exercise is *not* dancing: music is rhythm, rhythm is tension, but we want to *release* tension, so uncoordinated movement is vital.

2. Intentional Noise Garbage Exercise (INGE)

This is often introduced as a preparation for the later Intentional Verbalising Exercises. It fits neatly with the Motor Garbage Exercise, as both can be practised together. Many clients confess to feeling a bit silly with this one at first! These inhibitions will disappear in time, along with the tension.

It might be used:

- For relief of throat tension or tight breathing before speaking or singing
- Before interviews or presentations when it is important to express yourself clearly
- When experiencing difficulty in releasing emotions
- To loosen inhibitions imposed by education or society.

The INGE mimics the natural way in which children are able to make all sorts of noises that are not structured language, but are uninhibited and give release of tension.

The exercise consists of allowing yourself to indulge in making all those weird noises you were forbidden to make as a child. Play with your vocal cords, making any noise you wish: grunt, groan, blow 'raspberries', whatever. No words are used: the purpose of this exercise is 'sound' from within, nothing intellectual. Remember that the name of this is 'Noise' Garbage.

The secret is not to take yourself at all seriously. However, sometimes this exercise can lead to feelings of wanting to be angry (perhaps wanting to shout) or wanting to cry. If this happens, let it — allow your subconscious to release whatever it needs to.

This exercise takes anything from five seconds to five or ten minutes. Have as many breaks as you like, but give yourself sufficient time to feel relief. You can't do this exercise wrong. The only mistake is being caught doing it!

Often those who could most benefit from these exercises find them the hardest to do and it may take time and a gentle approach to become familiar with them.

Example

> A woman who often found it difficult to think of the right words
> 'in the heat of the moment' found a new ability to speak more
> fluently. Her self-confidence grew as a result.

THE PRINCIPLES AND BACKGROUND OF OFF-LOADING USING VERBALISATION

When the brain needs to off-load, it does so with words. We spontaneously off-load our feelings, often at inappropriate times. This might be stimulated by overload ('the last straw'), such as during an argument when all kinds of past issues are dragged up, which are irrelevant to the situation. Road rage is always an inappropriate response — probably reflective of overflowing levels of anger. Similarly with fear — perhaps you have experienced a near-miss on the motorway, or witnessed an accident. The natural inclination is to tell someone. This eases the fright and we go on telling people we meet until the fright lessens.

Expressing feelings verbally has a distinctly different effect from thinking about them. Thinking encourages them to fester — going round and round unceasingly. When we speak our feelings out loud, they are released, and their potency diminished. Repetition of this process increases the effectiveness of the release.

THE INTENTIONAL VERBALISATION EXERCISES

The Intentional Verbalisation Exercises are introduced around the fourth or fifth week of the course, when we have allowed the autogenic process to get established. At this stage, or before, there may be signs emerging that off-loading is beginning to occur in the Standard Exercises. This may be evident to your therapist long before it is to you, perhaps even from the initial assessment interview. Signs can show during observation of class exercises and from reading the training diary.

It is important for you to follow the therapist's instructions and, if necessary, keep in close contact while learning how to off-load.

Technical errors can render practice ineffectual or uncomfortable. Once you start working with these exercises, help and advice is always available from your therapist.

SEPARATION FROM AUTOGENIC EXERCISES

It is important to leave time between Intentional Verbalisation and Autogenic Exercises. In the first few practices, emotional material may not be cleared from the system effectively, and, if you do an Autogenic Exercise too soon afterwards, this might lead to a disturbance of it. It is also important that the effects of the Standard Exercises have worn off before off-loading is attempted. So, initially, it is recommended to leave at least one hour between Standard AT Exercises and Intentional Exercises. You will never use an AT posture when practising Intentional Verbalisation Exercises, so that inappropriate association with relaxation is avoided.

You will need to leave some time after the verbalisation before going to sleep. If the exercise is incomplete, the system needs a little time to settle down, or it may continue to discharge material in disturbing dreams.

SETTING UP INTENTIONAL VERBALISATION EXERCISES

You should not practise these exercises if you might feel inhibited by the thought of being overheard or interrupted. You may need the co-operation of family to be able to arrange time and space for your practice. The car may be a good place as long as it is stationary. Verbalisation exercises should not be done while driving, and time should be allowed to recover afterwards. You may choose to do these exercises under a duvet, to increase privacy. Playing loud music or doing the vacuuming will help to mask any noise.

You might plan two or three practice sessions per week to begin with. As things progress, you may need more or less time than this. As time goes on, you will know when you need to do an Intentional Verbalisation Exercise — your ability to spot the signs that it is needed comes with experience. If you are feeling distressed or agitated, it is sometimes more appropriate to do an

Intentional Exercise instead of an autogenic one.

When using these exercises for the first time, they can feel quite scary. Usually this is simply because of the unfamiliarity of them. We have learned to suppress our natural impulses so it may take a few attempts before we feel easy about them — even in private. Or we may feel that there is so much buried that we could be overwhelmed. These exercises are done when you are alone, so no one will interfere, and your defence mechanisms remain intact. Your therapist will show you how to limit the rate of release. You are not expected to revisit all of your life's past traumas — just enough to restore a balance.

Example

Miranda, aged 75 years, suffered sleep problems, extreme anxiety and physical fatigue. She had had a difficult childhood as a German Jew, and had had many traumatic episodes in her life since. One might imagine that the prospect of working on all this material at this stage in her life would have been too daunting to embark upon. On the contrary, Miranda relished the opportunity to release her feelings, and, after just two long sessions, she gained enormous relief. Subsequent anger exercises were of short duration and focused on current issues.

With persistence and the guidance of the therapist, great relief and profound beneficial changes can come from the use of these exercises.

3. Intentional Verbalisation of Aggression Exercise (IVAgg)

In today's society we see a great deal of inappropriate displays of anger, most of which are socially unacceptable. We cannot deal with all possibilities of global anger in this book, or indeed in all our lives. We can deal only with what confronts us as individuals in any given situation.

In our own lives we might give vent to our feelings of anger, and wish we hadn't. The aftermath of such expression can leave those around us hurt or uncomfortable, and ourselves guilty and feeling alienated. We can get caught between all-exploding rage (provoking guilt and shame) and suppression of all feelings (denial of anger). The letter reflects our efforts to be socially acceptable. We can learn to be afraid of anger, giving rise to non-specific anxiety. Those people who claim never to be angry are very likely learning AT in order to cope with their free-floating anxiety feelings.

However, it is worth considering anger as a valuable and positive emotion. It is a natural emotion of self-preservation — without anger we could not defend our loved ones or ourselves. It is an emotion about justice, or lack of it. Think of any campaign devoted to claiming human rights — the motivating force behind it will be anger.

The provocation to feel angry, annoyed, frustrated or irritated is all around, and the impulses are frequently triggered. Usually we will hold back on these impulses. Not to do that could mean destruction: of our jobs, relationships, etc., so we rightly use our suppression skills. But if we never allow ourselves to express that anger, the impulses are not discharged, but are stored within the body, as mentioned previously. This often gives rise to symptoms which may include irritability; left chest pain; abdominal discomfort; back pain; headaches; restlessness; fatigue. Even haemorrhoids (piles) may be a sign of repressed anger. This could be precipitated by constipation, itself a sign that the person may not be letting go (literally) of their 'rubbish'.

Once we have learned to deal effectively with our anger, we will be able to eliminate those symptoms, and prevent their recurrence. It stands to reason that fatigue and tiredness respond really well when anger is released — it takes a lot of energy to 'keep it down'. Release the old anger, and you will reclaim that energy for your own life.

The Intentional Verbalisation of Aggression allows for release of accumulated distressing material in a controlled environment.

It is not unusual to feel guilty or fearful as you first use this exercise, so remember: it is a technical cleaning exercise that will be of benefit to you and will improve relationships with those around you.

The purpose of this exercise is to teach us that anger is a normal, natural and necessary emotion. As you allow yourself to experience and express your anger safely, it will no longer be so distressing, either to yourself or to others.

You may find that during an anger exercise the focus of it changes. Feel free to move to another topic, explore any that emerge. This is why it is important to have considered all possible scenarios if incomplete off-loading is to be avoided. As you express your anger about the demands made on you by your boss, for instance, you may spontaneously switch your focus to your children, also making demands on you. Focusing on our children may feel unacceptable, but hold on to the reason for doing this. You are not getting angry with them, you are allowing yourself to release angry feelings which you have been harbouring — to the detriment of your well-being.

STRUCTURE OF THE INTENTIONAL VERBALISATION OF AGGRESSION EXERCISE

At the beginning, it is often helpful to make a list of people, events, situations which have triggered feelings of anger — both current and in the past. You will use this as a focus for your anger exercises. Allow yourself to include your nearest and dearest; yourself; those who have died; even your God.

The exercise is done in privacy and safety, by selecting a topic/person from the list. The 'target' may be imagined sitting in an empty chair, while you remain standing or sitting in a non-autogenic posture. To begin with, you can prime yourself with repetition of your usual swear words. These may be as strong as the 'F-word' or as mild as 'bother' — whatever you feel comfortable with. As you begin to focus on your target, the repetition of a phrase might be used. It is repeated over and over, out loud. For example, 'You silly cow', 'I hate the bastard', 'you make me so angry', etc. This is continued for as long as possible, letting it fade away to a murmur after a few minutes, or when the words become meaningless. If another phrase emerges, it is repeated in the same way, and so on. You will learn to be open to whatever thoughts come to your mind, *and feel free to express them*. Doing this will eventually feel natural. Continue to express your anger out loud until you feel 'emptied out'.

This may develop into (or you may choose to use) a monologue or one-sided tirade, telling the subject exactly what you think of them or describing what you wish would happen to them. It is very important that you do not stop in mid-flow. If you have managed to keep going for only a minute or so, don't give up — start again, as it may be that your usual inhibitions have kicked in to stop you. Any physical movement or activity that feels natural, such as hitting a pillow with your fist or a rolled-up magazine can accompany this. You may even feel like 'strangling' a towel! The mind will soon learn what is expected of it, and the process will become natural and spontaneous, with a feeling of conclusion and relief.

Any language which helps to express anger is excellent. Swearing is a wonderful aid to off-loading, but only if you are comfortable with it — if not, don't try it. It is only when these words are used in public that they are offensive.

If you work up 'a good head of steam' in your anger exercise, you might find yourself shouting and even screaming, or using wordless grunts. You will work through your anger faster if this happens. However, all Intentional Verbalisation Exercises should be kept within the bounds of comfort, so if you prefer to use dramatic stage whispers, or simply your normal speaking voice, that's fine.

Make sure that you keep the expression out loud — that you do not lapse into silent thoughts. We all know about those imaginary conversations which never resolve. In fact, they serve to encourage the angry thoughts to fester, compounding their damaging effect.

If you experience any anxiety or fear during the exercise, this should be allowed expression — similarly with crying or sadness which may occur.

WRITING

Sometimes it is difficult to find the right setting for out-loud work, so you can write down all your angry thoughts in a letter. Make sure that this is completely unstructured. The letter should not be a carefully reasoned argument — this will not express your anger. Use newspaper or scrap paper and an old ball-point, and let yourself 'stab' your target in your rage. You can help practise verbalisation by speaking as you write. *Do not send it!* Tear it up or burn it.

The length of a session will range from fifteen minutes to seventy-five minutes. It is important to continue until you feel that 'everything is out for now', and that there is nothing more to say for the moment.

If you finish too soon, you may experience increased irritability, moodiness and onset of headaches. *This is an indication to do another exercise at the earliest opportunity.* It does **not** mean that IVAgg is unsuitable for you or not working — quite the reverse. Another sign that you need to return to the IVAgg is if you find that passive concentration has deteriorated in subsequent autogenic Standard Exercises.

TECHNICAL ERROR
Do not off-load in person at the target of the exercise.

SUMMARY

Go as far as you are able without distress. Start gently — get used to the sound of your own voice alone in a room. As you gain confidence, you may want to shout, although this is not necessary. Do it only if you are certain that you are alone.

If you are interrupted or you are uncertain about when to stop, clench your fists and bend your arms sharply up to your shoulders, then have a good stretch. This will help you to break the mood quickly.

This is an exercise about you and your feelings — no judgement on what is right or wrong about them.

MEASURING LEVELS OF ANGER

Before considering this exercise, it is sometimes helpful to have an indication of the level of anger that may have accumulated. This can be done by keeping a chart of the daily frustrations, irritations and episodes of anger that are experienced. How often and how severely these events are experienced is a reflection of how much material we already have stored away.

It can be seen from the following example (Figure 5) that, over a very short time, although the triggers do not go away, the frequency and the severity of the response are greatly diminished. This would happen gradually with the use of the Standard Exercises but the process is greatly speeded up when Intentional Verbalisation of Aggression exercises are used.

The chart is filled in over the first week. As your list grows, you will write next to each item the intensity score. This is the level of anger you feel about it (e.g. frustration, mild irritation, annoyance, fury, outrage). You will also record the estimated frequency over one month (thirty days). These are then multiplied together to form the *activation score*. Your list may also be useful in picking out special problem areas where you might need to learn new ways of dealing with situations, people or incidents.

At the end of the course, the chart is reviewed. The intensity and frequency are re-assessed and multiplied to create the new activation score for each item. These are totalled to give an overall picture of levels of anger.

If Intentional Verbalisation of Aggression exercises have been used, it is very likely the scores have greatly reduced, often representing a freeing up of symptoms and a release of energy.

Figure 5: Chart Adapted from Dr Luthe's Workshop Notes of 1982
Prohomeostatic Aggression Control Inventory

	Name: Joan (age 44; high b/p)			Date Start of Course	Date End of Course
ITEM	INVENTORY (Situations, stimuli)	Intensity 1–5*	Frequency (no. of times per month)	Frequency multiplied by intensity	New frequency multiplied by new intensity
1	Children arguing	3	30	90	0
2	Untidiness	3	60	180	5
3	Rude shop assistants	3	4	12	0
4	Traffic gridlock	4	20	80	5
5	Computer — mind of its own	3	90	270	10
6	Cats	2	30	60	0
7	Car alarms at night	4	10	40	5
8	Thoughtless drivers	3	20	60	0
9	Things breaking down	3	10	30	2
10	Telephone cold calling	2	30	60	5
11	Work colleagues not working	3	30	90	0
12	Queuing	3	5	15	0
13	Mother's interference	3	10	30	2
14	Dan not helping	3	10	30	0
			TOTAL	1,047	34

* Intensity of anger feeling

1 = slight (a bit annoyed)

2 = somewhat (clearly irritated)

3 = moderate (somewhat angered)

4 = strong (enraged, exasperated)

5 = very strong (infuriated, loss of control)

CRYING AND GRIEF

Crying is natural. Children and babies are very good at it. Women are supposedly 'better at it' than men. However, we often associate crying with being 'weak' or 'giving in to emotion'. Or, we simply don't want to feel so bad that we have to cry. So we deny the need, suppress this natural response, even when we shouldn't. But we can also cry because we feel moved; because we are over-joyed; because we are relieved — then we may allow it because it feels more acceptable. Mostly, we recognise that crying is a good release. (When did you ever hear someone refer to 'a bad cry'?)

Yet still we do not cry enough. Our conditioning says that we are 'good' and 'brave' when we do *not* cry. Boys are 'sissy' if they cry. Girls are sneered at because they supposedly 'turn on the tears' to get their own way. Western society does not often encourage an open display of tears.

However, human beings are born with the extraordinary ability to influence their pain mechanism by switching on the crying mechanism to help their pain on its way; to work it out or through. A baby's crying brings the mother rushing to relieve it. Then, as the child grows, crying becomes less and less acceptable. We try to protect others by *not* crying (at funerals or during bereavement). Even when we do cry a little, we feel that this 'makes things worse'. The mind and body become adept at deceiving themselves, and it is likely that we all suppress our crying to a far greater extent than we realise.

It is not uncommon to find that, such is the resistance to cry-ing, we have become unaware of the need to cry, until the development of certain psychosomatic symptoms (see Chapter 7) which may lead us to think that we are ill. These Crying-Need Symptoms are indications that we have suppressed our need to cry.

Our reasoning does not usually allow us to accept a symptom of purely emotional origin. So much of our way of operating in the twenty-first century depends on finding answers (curing or reducing symptoms), that we unwittingly dismiss an idea such as generalised crying need. We do not need to have anything current to 'cry about' when faced with crying-need symptoms. These symptoms can build up over a period of years when we have long forgotten the original reason to cry.

GRIEF

Grief is usually associated with bereavement when a person dies. It is a state of feeling which is about loss, usually accompanied by sadness. Grief registers as pain. We hurt. Physical and emotional pain occurs many times throughout our lives. All the ordinary changes that we undergo in life involve loss and a degree of grief for what has gone before. But we do not always perceive grief in a normal life event. A child starting school needs to grieve for the loss of their previous life (we call it 'getting used to school', but surely it's really grief). Getting married, although presumably a positive event, needs a period of adjustment, but how often is this perceived and recognised as grief for the loss of the single life?

Luthe's research, linking crying-need symptoms with the use of Crying Exercises, did not reach a publishable stage before he died in 1985. Certainly, his ideas are controversial in some quarters, but any autogenic therapist will testify to the astonishing effect of symptom-relief when their clients use the Intentional Crying Exercise. There is an inevitable logic about these symptoms and their relief which is truly holistic — attending to the body, mind and spirit.

Have a look at the Crying Need Indications (symptoms) in Figure 6, and try to assess a rough percentage which you identify in yourself.

Have you noticed yourself sneezing for no apparent reason? Perhaps it lasts for a couple of hours, and then stops as mysteriously as it started.

When you do cry, how often have you stopped after a short while, because you are aware of a frontal headache or pressure (in your forehead)? You will stop crying 'because it makes my head hurt'. *But that is just the reason that you need to continue crying.* The forehead and sinuses are obvious places for the crying need to register — almost as the repository for unshed tears. If you suffer from 'chronic rhinitis', or 'post-nasal drip', you will probably be told it is an allergic response, and you may be prescribed a chemical agent to 'dry it up'. How about doing Crying Exercises to clear up your own 'allergy', by clearing out the old crying need?

The sob is an important part of crying, but when we do cry, more often than not we cry silently, allowing tears to run down the face, and 'stuffing the pillow in the mouth' in order not to be heard. However, the sound and movement of the sob are an integral part of the crying mechanism, allowing strong movements in the lower part of the lungs, and release of sound. This sound can be a wail or moaning. When it is accompanied by the particular lung movements of the sob, it comes in short sharp bursts. When the sob is suppressed, we experience pain, or a 'lump in the throat'. If you stop yourself crying, observe how tense your muscles become, in your efforts to stop the crying movement in the body. This too explains the many crying-need symptoms.

THE CRYING NEED SUPPRESSED IS THE GRIMACE DENIED

Where did the expression 'stiff upper lip' come from? It may have originated in the First World War, when soldiers, coping with the grief and loss of their friends, along with their personal fears, had to 'soldier on', suppressing the need to cry, in order to cope. If they felt the tell-tale sign of the face wanting to crumple into the 'crying grimace', the lip would begin to quiver. Biting the lip, or stretching it, would stop the tremble, and successfully keep tears and crying at bay. Similarly, other symptoms can appear for the same reason, such as twitching muscles around the eyes and mouth.

TWO SIDES OF A COIN: CRYING AND LAUGHING

When you think about laughing, it is always associated with a good feeling. Laughter is fun: we can smile at the memory of a good joke; we can laugh out loud even when no one else is around. Research has shown that laughter is 'good medicine'. We love 'a good old belly-laugh'. We feel our spirits are lifted, recognising that humour is a wonderful defuser of irritation.

But what about those people who laugh 'too much', making jokes out of everything? Do you feel that such a person does not listen to you because they are too busy giving the witty response? They probably add a good dose of cynicism to every conversation.

Perhaps the cynics are also displaying a crying need — although they would hotly deny it. Their defence will be that humour is good — it lightens the mood. It cheers everyone up. But does it — always? The cynic may have got into this unconscious habit as a result of denying expression of feeling in the past. This kind of behaviour can be very frustrating for others, as opinions and requests are dismissed or trivialised. The office clown is not always as popular as they think.

To laugh and to cry are very similar in their physical mechanisms. Look in the mirror and experiment: the face uses muscles to stretch the mouth in a smile, corners up, showing teeth and narrowing the eyes. The crying grimace also features a stretched mouth, but the corners are down: teeth show, eyes narrow. Even the sound of laughter is similar to the sound of crying: short sharp emissions through the vocal cords from the diaphragm, as the lungs push the air through. Crying is usually accompanied by tears — laughter can also involve tears. We all know that bizarre feeling when we have been in paroxysms, perhaps of 'hysterical', 'uncontrollable' laughter, at something which no longer feels funny, and, before we know it, we are crying. In this scenario we may not even recognise what it is we are crying about, but we can view this as the body's need to grab the opportunity for emotional release.

Figure 6: Indications for Intentional Crying Exercise (from Luthe workshop notes 1982)

Crying-Need Symptoms

Examples of Individually Variable crying-need symptoms which subside after sufficient crying has occurred:

1. Activation of Depressive Dynamics
No interest, no initiative, feelings of frustration, feelings of being 'fed up', social withdrawal, fatigue, tiredness

---

2. Activation of Anxiety Dynamics
Feeling more apprehensive than usual, increased impatience, feelings of insecurity, enhanced phobic reactions

3. Activation of Aggressive Dynamics
Irritability, destructive actions or verbal reactions, feelings of rejection, tendency to disturb others, trouble-making for oneself and others (you know you shouldn't, but you can't help picking quarrels)

4. General Malaise
Feeling physically unwell, minor aches and pains, noticeable tension, minor respiratory and gastro-intestinal complaints, stuffy and runny nose (when you do not have a cold)

5. General Unexplained Aches and Pains
Pains and aches in upper and lower back, extremities, neck, chest; haemorrhoids; frontal headaches; pains in joints, bones, muscles

6. Activation of Various Psycho-Physiologic (or allergic) Reactions
Skin problems, gastro-intestinal problems, discomfort in the eyes, nose, ears and throat, sinusitis, chronic catarrh, hay fever, bronchial asthma, swelling of joints, essential bursitis (swelling and fluid in a joint unexplained by injury), frequent need to urinate (sometimes described as 'because of nerves'), vaginal discharge

7. Activation of Motor Phenomena Related to Crying
Irritating dry cough, hoarseness, fading voice, sneezing, frequent yawning, frequent swallowing, sighing, facial tics, fluttering eyelids, trembling of lips, twitching of perioral muscles (around mouth), 'artificial' laughing, irregular respiration

8. Variable Awareness of Need for Crying
The need to cry repeatedly suppressed or repressed, unawareness of need to cry, associative resistance (conditioning/social culture), wishing to cry but unable to do so

Additional symptoms we have frequently observed are: pressure round the forehead and eyes; pain between the shoulder blades; lump in the throat; sore or itching eyes and nose; sad dreams.

The Intentional Crying Exercise allows the physical crying mechanism to influence the pain mechanism and heal the pain.

4. INTENTIONAL CRYING EXERCISE (ICE)

This exercise once again mimics the system's natural response — this time using the movements and sounds related to crying, without necessarily shedding tears. The Crying Exercise is a technical cleaning exercise to off-load unexpressed effects of pain. It is not necessary to engage in sadness. You can do the job by simulating the physical motions of crying, using the muscles of deep sobbing. These include the abdominal and chest muscles, sometimes with shoulder and arm movements. Moaning and sobbing sounds are made. This will sometimes tip you into real crying — give yourself permission and go along with it until conclusion.

A private place to practise is important, so that you are not inhibited. A few minutes are often sufficient to clear the system of current material. However, as the AT process develops, there may be a need to do more.

The exercise is done by pretending to act the part of someone who is crying bitterly about some personal loss. All the gestures of real crying are used: facial expressions, shoulders heaving, sobbing noises. This is continued for as long as can comfortably be managed. For some people, this will be only a few minutes, and 'little and often' may be the rule for them. Others may achieve twenty minutes comfortably. It is important that any real crying which emerges be allowed the opportunity to work its course.

DR LUTHE SUGGESTS

1 Tears are a luxury. Technical crying does **not** require 'production' of real tears. (Do not chop onions to make them!)
2 Do not artificially 'pump up' painful memories, imagine sad events, or use evocative music to produce sad feelings.

3 Do not practise ICE in insecure circumstances (such as when you may be disturbed — by children, pets, phone, etc.)

4 Warn the family; try practising under a duvet or blankets, or in the shower; put the radio on, or do the hoovering to drown out the sound.

Our experience says that there are many different ways of carrying out a Crying Exercise. If, when you start, sad memories do occur, simply allow yourself to go along with them, and indulge in your crying response. The important thing is to get going on it in any way you can. (However, don't use imaginary events to stimulate crying.) Some people speak their grief, finding it easier to talk about sadness and loss than do the simulated crying straightaway. This type of talking might lead into crying, simulated or real.

This exercise feels and seems quite alien and awkward at first. Feeling 'stupid' is the most likely result until you are used to it. Try short bursts until you feel more familiar with sustaining longer exercises. Once you have overcome your inhibition, you can start to congratulate yourself, especially when you notice the reduction of symptoms.

Not Doing Enough

If your crying exercise is finished too soon, your crying inhibition is coming into play, and you may feel rather worse. As a result, some of the crying-need symptoms may re-appear.

This is an indication to do another exercise at the earliest opportunity. It does **not** mean that ICE is unsuitable for you or not working — quite the reverse. Try doing short Crying Exercises (little and often), to help the release process. You need to give your system an opportunity to work through that, and towards a more continuous flow.

Using this exercise, you can discover how quickly irritating symptoms can disappear.

Case 1 — Robert (frontal headaches)

Robert was a man in his mid-fifties, 'something high-powered' in the City. His sole reason for learning AT was his suffering from severe frontal headaches. He had consulted with his GP and specialists, and had had every investigation possible. He had used acupuncture, chiropractic, osteopathy, medical herbs. These had helped, but not permanently. He told his AT therapist, 'You are my last resort'. From his history the therapist recognised his headaches as a possible crying need, and Robert complained after two weeks of the course that his headaches were generally worse — and more severe during AT exercises. The ICE was introduced in the third week. The following week, Robert arrived beaming. He had practised the ICE on three occasions and his headaches were beginning to improve. The following week he reported daily ICE, and after four days his headache disappeared. His head stayed clear while practising AT exercises. He continued ICE once daily, and AT three times daily, and there were no further reports of headaches. He said that he would continue his ICE because it was easy to practise for one minute every morning while cleaning his teeth!

Robert had no need to know what he was crying about. The ICE simply exercises the mechanism of the body to clear out the crying need. Just *do* it — and the benefits arrive.

Case 2 — George (undiagnosed abdominal pain)

George was a usually fit 35-year-old married man who had been off work for four months with severe, but undiagnosed, abdominal pain. He had been recommended for AT by his GP — as a means to help him cope with his condition, at least, if not find a cure. From his history and the description of the pain, and the sense of despair about it, his AT therapist knew

---

that ICE would play an important part in his recovery. When asked about his crying 'habits', George replied that, yes, his symptoms had provoked him to crying at times. Further questioning elicited that his crying had been short-lived — he'd pulled himself together for the sake of his wife and family. He didn't want to feel that his condition had caused him to feel such emotional extremes. But his body was literally 'crying out'. Other symptoms showed it too: he was constantly irritable and crotchety with his family; he suffered anxiety and occasional panics. He described his 'relapses' as depressing, and he withdrew from social contact. During the first two weeks of the course, his symptoms came and went, but in the third week he described the pain as so bad that he felt tearful. When asked if he had cried, he vehemently denied it.

His therapist wondered whether he needed to express anger rather than crying, but he did not fully engage with the Intentional Anger exercises ('It makes me feel sad'.) At the sixth session, he described extreme tiredness and exhaustion during the week. At the seventh session, he described finding new energy — doing some DIY and pacing himself. He did not experience his usual pain after it. Then he told how he had practised ICE several times during the week — for five or ten minutes each time. His therapist urged him to use the ICE as often as he could — even to the extent of sacrificing one of his daily autogenic exercises if necessary. By the end of the course, George reported that he had been completely pain-free for several days, and six weeks later he was back at work.

ICE played a major part in this, and, in addition, George reported that his anxiety about his illness was very much reduced. The sheer expression of feeling had had a really positive effect on his whole outlook. Add to that his reported increase in creativity, and plans to patent some of his ideas, and you can see that AT certainly did its job!

ANXIETY

Worry, anxiety and fear are protective emotions. Their original purpose was to prevent us from rushing headlong into dangerous situations. The caveman needed these responses for survival. But he also knew, instinctively, how to rest, recover and recuperate. In our modern society we are bombarded with information, demands and expectations. We need to perform to hold down our jobs — we keep on going, ignoring signals from our minds and bodies until they are overwhelming. A major panic attack might stop us in our tracks, giving a sharp warning that all is not well within.

In addition, our anxiety habits are topped up by the media's propensity to feed us negative material. Children are over-protected because of parents' fears for them — they grow up without learning that anxiety is OK, that it can be used to learn from and that there are ways to find solutions.

The brain does not find it easy to distinguish what *has* happened from what *might* happen (i.e. the reality versus imagination). We can originate our own anxiety entirely from imagination. Anxious thinking can be picked up from parents at an early age, and may become a habit. A constant state of worry can occur, with no obvious focal point. This is known as free-floating anxiety (or 'non-specific anxiety') and comes from an accumulation of suppressed fear. (*'If I have nothing to worry about, I worry until I have found something to worry about.'*)

As we have seen with other unexpressed emotion, unexplained physical and psychological symptoms can also occur with repressed anxiety. These symptoms may include: tiredness; headaches; nausea; palpitations; hyperventilation; dizziness; restlessness; panic attacks; disturbing dreams; early waking; depression; muscle tension; phobias; digestive problems.

5. INTENTIONAL VERBALISATION OF ANXIETY EXERCISE (IVANX)

There is a cultural reluctance to admit to our fears, even to ourselves, and it is often thought that saying our fears out loud increases them, or provokes a feared event. This is not the case. This exercise allows the discharge of an accumulation of unexpressed anxiety. Consider how you naturally deal with a situation that has frightened you — you speak about it to the next person you meet, and continue to tell people until you start to feel better.

VERBAL REPETITION OF FEAR CAN HELP TO DISCHARGE IT
This exercise mimics our natural behaviour by encouraging repetition of a phrase or a series of phrases about our fears. The task is to give the brain the opportunity to off-load feelings of anxiety and fear in a safe setting, away from the triggers which cause the feelings. *(Do not do your IVAnx exercise about your fear of flying while sitting on the plane waiting for takeoff! You should have done plenty, daily, for about three weeks before the flight. A Standard Autogenic Exercise will be best on the plane.)* It is a technical cleaning exercise — you may or may not encounter real anxiety feelings while doing it.

ANXIETY AS A MASK
Emotions are complex and not always easily recognised. It is common for feelings of anxiety to originate from unexpressed anger or pain, hurt and loss. The presence of free-floating, non-specific anxiety without a focus may well indicate this. If we have unwittingly suppressed anger or crying, we may have converted the feeling to one of anxiety — as though we are afraid of our feelings.

PRELIMINARY ASSESSMENTS
Before starting the exercise, it may be helpful to consider the levels of anxiety in your life by making a list of your anxieties: people, situations, etc. You will end up with a comprehensive list, which in itself can be a help — overwhelming feelings can be significantly reduced just by being acknowledged on paper. This is different from the Anxiety Control Inventory which deals with current triggers, although the contents may be similar.

The exercise is done by walking about or sitting in a non-autogenic posture. A topic or focus is taken from the list, and verbalisation about it takes place **out loud** (e.g. 'I am afraid'; 'I'm worried'; 'I don't want to go'; 'I am afraid to die'; 'I am afraid of making a fool of myself'.) Each phrase is repeated over and over until it has been repeated enough. At this point, clear speech changes to mumbling and then to silence. After a period of silence, another phrase comes to mind and is repeated in the same way. This is kept going for as long as possible, with new phrases being introduced as they occur to you, until you reach a point of calm. It is important to wait during a pause to be certain that no new phrase is going to come up before finishing.

It may be preferable to use a monologue: tell yourself out loud in detail what is worrying you. Give yourself plenty of time to explore, identify and release your worries and fears until you reach a point of calm. You may need a few brief breaks during a session.

Make sure that you continue for long enough. Ending the exercise too early can lead to side effects such as irritability, moodiness, anxiety or headache. If such side effects should occur, this is an indication that there is more to come, and you should continue at the earliest opportunity.

It is a technical error to do this silently. You will reinforce and increase your anxiety if you do not speak it out loud.

Five to fifteen minutes will usually be enough to provide satisfactory relief. If not, revisit the exercise at another time.

Again, to achieve the privacy you need, try turning on the television or radio, sitting in your car, muffling your voice with a pillow, running the bath, or burying yourself under the duvet.

MEASURING LEVELS OF ANXIETY
As with the Intentional Verbalisation of Aggression Exercise, it can be useful to measure the current level of day-to-day anxiety that is being experienced, as a reflection of accumulated material.

The chart (Figure 7) is recorded and scored as before. As you re-assess, you will see that although many of the triggers may still be present, the severity of the response is much reduced. This is again reflected in a reduction of symptoms and a release of energy.

Figure 7: Chart Adapted from Dr Luthe's Workshop Notes of 1982 Prohomeostatic Anxiety Control Inventory

	Name: Andrew (age 38; teacher)			Date Start of Course	Date End of Course
ITEM	INVENTORY (Situations, stimuli)	Intensity 1–5★	Frequency (no. of times per month)	Frequency multiplied by intensity	New frequency multiplied by new intensity
1	Car breaking down	4	20	80	5
2	Motorway in the rain at night	4	10	40	10
3	Meeting deadlines at work	4	30	120	30
4	Official school inspection next year	4	120	480	5
5	Meeting parents at school	4	60	240	0
6	My course work	3	30	90	5
7	Overdraft	3	30	90	0
8	Child's health	4	30	120	10
9	Wife's health	3	30	90	5
10	Own health	3	60	180	5
11	Child's progress at school	3	15	45	0
12	House repairs	2	15	30	0
13	Arguments with my wife	4	60	240	5
14	The news	2	60	120	5
15	My parents	2	10	20	0
			TOTAL	1,955	80

★ Intensity of anxiety feeling

1 = uneasy (a bit apprehensive)

2 = clearly worried/anxious

3 = rising anxiety

4 = quite frightened, scared

5 = panic, badly frightened

SUMMARY

When you have completed a good-quality and effective off-loading exercise, you will feel better and find that the quality of passive concentration in subsequent Standard Exercises improves. So, Intentional Verbalisation Exercises do a great deal to improve and enhance your autogenic experience.

If the Intentional Verbalisation Exercises are to be of value, they must offer the system the opportunity to discharge a variety of suppressed material. Often, one of the exercises becomes favourite, to the neglect of the others. It may be that there is a reluctance to visit potentially painful areas; or you may not recognise the need after years of suppression.

Not everyone will take to the Intentional Off-loading Exercises. This may be because they do not recognise the need, and the idea is too alien to accept. If clients are honest with themselves in examining their responses to life events, it is hoped that they will come to recognise the potential value of this work.

If, at first, you are resistant to these exercises, you may become convinced of their efficacy as you experience their use, and overcome some of your training problems, or witness the success of others in the training group. Initially, you may fear 'lifting the lid' on uncomfortable material, or you may consider there is too much material to be dealt with. Or your response might be: 'I only came to lower my blood pressure, and what has emotion to do with that?' (Both authors can give examples of how using IVAgg has helped to bring about a reduction in high blood pressure.)

If the time is not 'right' now, it may come, and these techniques can be helpful in the future. However, they do take practice, so it is recommended that you give them a go. If there are any difficulties, the therapist can help.

There is no doubt that the benefits of persisting and overcoming resistance are great. You may well avoid further time-consuming and expensive therapy.

6. INTENTIONAL VOMITING EXERCISE

This exercise may not be routinely introduced as part of an AT course, but it is useful in some circumstances.

Consistent abdominal discomfort, feelings of nausea or a clearly experienced need to 'throw up' during an autogenic exercise are all possible indicators that this form of tension release is necessary.

Nausea often occurs as an emotional response — to bad news, for example. The body's instinctive response is to 'throw up' the feelings induced by the information, just as it might need to get rid of bad food. The nauseous feeling is caused by tension in the cardiac sphincter muscle connecting the oesophagus and stomach. This tension is released by practising the Intentional Vomiting Exercise.

A consistently suppressed need to vomit, or a fear of vomiting, can be an indication of the need for this exercise. There may be an old memory or fear of losing consciousness as the result of a past accident, which has inhibited vomiting. These can give rise to tensions which need to be off-loaded. Sometimes a vomiting need seems to be symbolically related to feelings described by the phrase 'I'm sick of such-and-such' or 'So-and-so makes me sick'.

This exercise is not suitable if you have problems with stomach or duodenal ulcer or hiatus hernia; you are pregnant; you suffer or have suffered from any form of eating disorder.

It is not necessary to rehearse this exercise. When you need it, just do it. It is over and done with very quickly, and there is absolutely no need to empty the stomach contents. The purpose is to initiate the vomiting reflex, simply exercising the muscles of stomach and oesophagus. Choose a secure setting (the bathroom) and initiate the vomiting reflex by simulating noises of being sick (or you can put your finger down your throat). Initiate the reflex several times.

You will know immediately when you have done enough. A feeling of relief occurs after three or four 'gags'. Sometimes several sessions are needed before the symptoms disappear completely.

CHAPTER 6

PERSONAL AND MOTIVATIONAL FORMULAE

Towards the end of the course, or at the very end, you will be give instruction on how to use personal or motivational formulae. Schultz developed this idea to enable the mind to capitalise on the work already achieved through the Standard Exercises. It is a very interesting stage of the process, which enables the individual to address a specific area for change and make a definite mark in breaking a habit or enhancing a particular aspect of their lives. In other settings these phrases are known as positive affirmations. So, as well as using it looking in the mirror, walking down the street and standing in queues, you will also be reinforcing its message in that optimum state — during autogenic exercises.

These formulae are special — for your own self only. Similar to the 'post-hypnotic suggestion' used in hypnosis, the aim is to plant the seed of an idea into your mind while it is engaged in the altered state of consciousness of AT. As long as you have found the right wording, you have every chance of making exciting and interesting changes to your life and well-being.

The key is to know what you want. Avoid making a shopping list of wonderful attributes you wish you had. No — the purpose of these is to enhance and encourage your acceptance of yourself. These phrases will have their individual profound meanings, and need to be structured carefully so that they will not be misinterpreted by the unconscious and give an unfavourable result! A good place to start is often to focus on some aspect of change in yourself, which you have already noticed during the course.

Personal and motivational formulae can be used for all kinds of problems, such as:

107

- Self-esteem
- Eating problems
- Smoking
- Concentration
- Memory
- Stuttering
- Insomnia
- Health
- Mood
- Relationships
- Performance.

These formulae are added to the Standard Exercises. They were originally known as intentional formulae, to differentiate them from Standard AT, because they carry a specific intent. However, they are now known as 'personal' or 'motivational', in order to distinguish them from the Intentional Exercises.

The exciting and varied possibilities for AT to add to its already comprehensive repertoire for healing and rebalance are endless. At the end of the course of Standard Exercises, the system is familiar with responding to its own inner voice, and passive concentration can be identified and maintained. So, it is a good next step to learn how to 'personalise' your AT. Here, the essence is not so much about allowing a spontaneous self-righting process, as about allowing an idea to flower through passive introduction to the subconscious.

PURPOSE OF THE PERSONAL FORMULA

The personal formula is usually concerned with influencing a change in personal attitude or behaviour. So, these formulae do carry an intent. You will need to work carefully to word the formula so that the same passive approach can be used as in the Standard Exercise.

Dr Klaus Thomas, Schultz's colleague at the Berlin Institute, has written several books on the subject of the personal formula — all in German unfortunately.

PLACING OF THE FORMULA

There are three options commonly used:

1. AFTER THE PEACE FORMULA

When you reach the end of the exercise, repeat your special phrase over and over. This gives an opportunity for quiet reflection/ meditation on it before closing. If you wish, you can repeat the Peace Formula again — to allow the 'no-thought' phase after it.

2. BEFORE THE PEACE FORMULA

If you prefer to end the exercise with the peace formula, place the personal formula after using the neck and shoulders formula. Repeat it several times. Then use the peace formula and allow yourself to slip into a no-thought place where profound healing and rebalancing takes place.

3. IN THE NEUTRAL STATE — THE 'NO-THOUGHT PHASE' (SEE CHAPTER 4)

At times you will find yourself in the Neutral State at any point during the exercise and this is also a good place to use the personal formula.

As you come to the realisation and recognition of the neutral state, you can slot your personal formula in. It doesn't matter where you got to in the exercise — drop your special formula in here. This is very much akin to planting the seed in fertile soil — the idea will take root more strongly than simply repeating the phrase while walking around town. Of course, you can do both.

Using the Personal Formulae in the Neutral State

The moment of awareness that this 'other place' has been reached (often with heaviness and warmth formulae or the breathing formula) is the exact moment where adding the personal formula will bring the greatest effect, as the mind and body are at their most receptive at this point. Use it several times. After this, you can close the exercise, or continue from a certain point, or just add the peace formula.

In some exercises the neutral state will occur easily. Other exercises will be a fairly routine go-through, in which case the personal formula can be placed at the very end, after the peace formula. It is important to remember that non-striving principles still apply. Do not try to find the neutral state. It will not happen through striving.

Only one formula is used to begin with. It is repeated several times, and a few minutes are spent meditating on its significance. Allow three to four weeks for the phrase to take effect. How long it takes depends on the size of the problem and your ability to reach the neutral state. Some changes take several months. A second related formula can be added after three to four weeks, but don't use more than two formulae at the same time.

CONSTRUCTING A PERSONAL FORMULA

The best formula is one which uses your own words. You will have been given clear guidelines on the structure of the formula, with some ideas of its format (a rhyming couplet, for example). Your therapist may help and guide you in constructing your phrase, but they may also stand back and leave it to you. You should have a lot of freedom to play around with ideas, bearing in mind that the guidelines are important, to maximise the potential of the idea. You should not feel too inhibited by the rules to experiment. On the other hand, if you pay no attention to how you construct your formula, you can bring about the opposite effect to what you intended.

You should have fun with this. The brain can allow a lot of creativity, within the basic idea of 'short, simple, positive, passive and present tense'.

GUIDELINES
1. Preparation
The personal and motivational formula is not a New Year's resolution — we all know what happens to those! The formula is a

real possibility, not just wishful thinking. It should be something for your own sake — not to please others.

It is useful first to make a list of the possibilities: 'What do I want to change?' For example,

- *I want to stop blushing.*
- *I want to cope better in interviews.*
- *I want a better job.*
- *I want to travel on the tube by myself.*

When you examine the list, you may find a common thread. In the above example, this may be about confidence. You might construct one formula which addresses all this, such as: '*I am calm and confident*' or '*I enjoy life's adventures*'.

Don't be too ambitious on Day 1. For example, if you have been a 40-a-day smoker for forty years, don't decide to give up as your first experience of using a personal formula. Most smokers don't succeed in giving up until they *want* to (more's the pity). So, if you put an unreasonable amount of pressure on yourself, your brain will object and let you down. Ask yourself about your relationship to cigarettes after using AT. You may have spontaneously cut down a bit.

Now, prepare the ground by finding out what it is that smoking does for you. So, if you are aware that you need to light up when you are tense and anxious, then a more innocuous phrase like 'I am calm and centred' will be a more appropriate start. See how you respond to that over a few weeks. Then you might use 'I am calm and centred without cigarettes'. When the time is right, you will be able to give up much more easily.

2. One Formula
Use only one personal formula at a time to start with.

3. A Second Formula
After three or four weeks, you may add another formula, perhaps by using the word 'and' to connect the two. Bear in mind that some changes will take several months to occur.

For example, '*I am calm and centred*' might become '*I am calm and centred and have plenty of time for everything*'.

4. Short and Simple

The formula should be short and simple. In general, a message is more readily accepted and more memorable if it is short.

However, as an exception, Dr Klaus Thomas cites the example of a 37-year-old lawyer who suffered from epilepsy and devised the following:

> Whenever a fit is approaching I lie down, sit down or stand still. I stop any activity and instruct a partner. Blood is streaming into my brain, where the arteries open. In the fit I lie down calmly, I do not talk, nor do I undertake anything. I only act when I am quite clear again. I do not give in, I hold on!

He often added:

> You need not be ashamed about the consequences of your being wounded. Brain scar is warmly flooded with blood.

Apparently this formula was most effective, reducing the number of epileptic fits from eight or more per month to an average of less than one, which was more easily managed — 'milder'. The man was able to resume his work.

Thomas points out that the formula did not adhere to any of the recommended rules, but the patient mastered it to the extent that it had become a part of his inner self. The result is much more important than the rules.

This example is most interesting because the man is clearly accepting the problem without trying to wish it away. He could have used 'My epilepsy is better'. Clearly this would be untrue. However, he focused on remaining calm and accepting in his attitude and behaviour while having a fit. And the fits reduced in frequency. (Was his epilepsy getting better?)

5. Present Tense

The formula is always in the present tense — 'My nails *are* long and strong', never 'I am *going to*' or 'I *will* stop biting my nails'.

6. Positive Statement

Always use a positive statement. It is well known that the brain is unable to accept a negative statement when it is in an altered state of consciousness. It needs intellect to help process the negative element. So, a positive statement reaches the unconscious immediately. The same principle applies when speed is needed. Think of a child running downhill. The parent shouts, 'Don't you fall over'. The child falls. The command 'fall over' has been absorbed before interpreting 'Don't' in connection with it. If the parent says, 'Take care', or 'Mind how you go', the child is allowed a far better chance to slow down without an accident.

Some negative statements are acceptable, as long as they carry a nonchalant, throw-away type of attitude. (See neutralising formulae, p. 117.)

7. Passive Phrase

The phrase should be passive. Avoid words such as 'want', 'ought', 'should', 'must'. These words could bring about a perversely opposite response: 'I might not'; 'Who says?' Too much pressure is suggested, or the feeling that a result is paramount. Our social conditioning might be making its mark here, in that most of us have been brought up to put our own wishes at the bottom of the heap. Phrases carrying words such as 'I allow myself' or 'I am' convey a feeling of gentle acceptance of the self, while giving the possibility of real and achievable change.

For example, '*I must do my AT twice a day*' becomes '*I allow myself regular AT exercises*' or simply '*I love my AT* '.

8. Acceptable Phrase

Make sure that the phrase is acceptable. You might be given ideas of what to use in your personal formula. Your therapist, for example, may think a certain phrase would be a good one for your asthma. But you might have a better one, as you know yourself better than anyone else. So, when your therapist suggests, '*My breathing flows*', and you feel as though you are drowning when you use it, clearly, it is wrong. As you explore the issues around your asthma, you may come up with very different ideas, which on the surface seem to bear no relation to breathing (for example, '*I love myself*'; '*I am in charge of my life*'; '*I am calm and confident*'). Try them — they will be more potent as they have come from *your* ruminations, not someone else's.

If you consistently forget what your personal formula is, or forget to use it, you are probably using words which do not adequately express your meaning. Adjust the formula, or drop it altogether for a while. You may find that the perfect words pop into your head one day without even thinking about them: the wonders of the right brain!

The personal formula is a gift — from you to you.

INCREASED EFFECTIVENESS

There are many ways to play around with words in order to find the right way to express the special message to the self. Dr Klaus Thomas writes of using rhyme and alliteration in ways that appeal to the creative side of ourselves. The secret is to create something that makes you feel good. It may make you smile with anticipation as you look forward to using it. It may even make you laugh. We all know how humour and laughter are not only a great healer, but they also help a learning process. So, involving all our positive feelings will bring about positive outcomes. The following are a few examples:

Personal and Motivational Formulae

Menacing Men Menace Me Not (for the woman afraid of walking home in the dark)
This uses alliteration in a very clever manner. Also, the strong syllable in the phrase is at the end of it. Its negative quality is delivered in such a positive style that it serves as a confidence booster.

Driving along with my passenger load
I'm calm and confident reading the road.
This was designed for a young man of 19, who had failed four of his allotted five attempts to pass his bus driving test. After some discussion as to the problem, it was suggested that he use the above phrase, and because it exactly described the difficulty, he accepted it immediately. (He passed his test!)

Sometimes, rather than search for new and exciting areas to change our lives, it is a good start to build on whatever has emerged so far from your AT. For example:

My Willingness to Work is Wonderful
This was suggested for the student who had already discovered that he could study with greater ease and sense of flow, without stopping every ten minutes for yet another cup of coffee. Here, he knew the phrase would be successful because he was familiar with the intended outcome. He achieved a 2:1 degree instead of his predicted 2:2.

Use the following to help the unconscious to absorb and enforce the message:

- Rhyme
- Rhythm
- Alliteration
- Humour.

The phrase may emerge in a slogan-like form. It may contain a joke appreciated only by you.

Sometimes a piece of music may spring to mind during an AT exercise. Allow it to run its course in the form of 'silent singing'. Perhaps it is a particular lyric which carries meaning, or the beauty of the tune itself. Use a piece of poetry, or a favourite quote from the bible, or any source that is inspirational to you.

Some therapists will encourage you to change the wording of a literary or religious source so that words like 'I', 'me' or 'my' are included. In the Standard Exercises you will have been using 'my' and 'I' as a routine, and the personal formula should follow this pattern, the reason being that you should keep in touch with your ego, maintaining an internal locus of control, rather than putting all your healing powers in the power of some other force or deity (external locus of control). Ask yourself, as you prepare a formula which implies that God will look after you, whether you are giving yourself enough choice/power in this.

Some therapists encourage their clients to retain a detachment alongside their passivity, and use the Standard Exercises without the personal article (no reference to 'my' and 'I'). In this case there is no reason to use it in the personal formula. Your acceptance of the Standard Exercises without 'my/I' will play the same part in the selection of your personal formula.

USE OF WORDS

Be aware of how you are using words. For example, someone suffering from panic attacks should avoid using the word 'panic' in their formula. We have found that in most cases it is better to avoid a key-word in the personal formula — it can put the system 'on alert'. When you are in a deeply relaxed state, is it really wise to use a word that could provoke the exact opposite?

Instead, ask yourself what you desire, and build up the positive. This will appeal to the psyche more than attempting to banish a negative feeling using the very key-word that might provoke it.

For example, rather than '*Panic leaves me*', try '*I love parties*' or '*I know my subject*' or '*Life is interesting*'.

Appropriate Wording
Always use wording appropriate for the meaning you require.

Example

> Sheila complained that her personal formula wasn't working. She had been using it for several months, so lack of perseverance wasn't the problem. She had chosen: 'I can release my anger'. She found that she was being snappy and irritable, picking quarrels, and being a general 'pain in the neck' (her words) — all the things she was trying to avoid. Further questioning revealed what she was aiming for: 'I wanted to let go — at last — stop carrying around all this anger which has been with me for years.' JB suggested that she might have used, 'I release myself from my anger', and this made absolute sense. Sheila changed at once — to good effect. However, JB did not miss the opportunity to encourage Sheila to use the Intentional Verbalisation of Aggression Exercise.

Spontaneous Selection of Formula

Dr Brian O'Donovan recommends a way of choosing a formula that allows the brain in the autogenic state to meditate on a word and allow the subconscious to construct its own wording. This should be done with as little conscious thought, or active concentration, as possible.

Select a word from the following:

Love	Peace
Joy	Harmony
Light	Tranquil
Quiet	Still
Pleasure	Health
Happiness	Vigour
Well-being	Strength

or find another of your own. Take your word with you into the AT exercise.

Close your eyes in an autogenic posture. Practise an autogenic exercise. After the peace formula stay in position at the end, and meditate on your chosen word. Stay with this until a phrase emerges. Then meditate on it for a while. Close.

THE GROUP FORMULA

Some therapists suggest encouraging the group to find a formula that echoes, reflects or summarises the work they have done together. Sometimes group members suggest a formula for each other. This can be very rewarding, as the creative, humorous mind of one person offers an idea to another. But we need to be sure that one group member isn't trying to wield their own power with clever suggestions. Be prepared to say 'No — that just isn't for me'.

For a group formula, your therapist will ask some leading questions, drawn from their observations, to provoke an idea or two, and will then leave it to the group.

If the group has been a harmonious one, with support and positive regard for each other, they will come up with some good ideas. Take a vote on which formula seems the best for that moment (maybe it focuses on the future, while using the present tense), and it will be used in the final group exercise.

TYPES OF PERSONAL FORMULA

Schultz and Luthe described five different types. For any formula there are cautions. Ask yourself how you feel about the style of words you have chosen. Do they make your heart sing? Do you feel a secret smile about them?

1. NEUTRALISING FORMULA

This type implies that something really doesn't matter, is not important. It usually applies to a situation or circumstance that causes anxiety or panic, and can neutralise the negative feeling associated with it. It is useful for the person who has become obsessive, to the detriment of their performance, or restriction of their lifestyle.

Examples

- *Crowds don't matter.*
- *Exams don't matter.*
- *Housework doesn't matter.*

The message gradually takes the pressure out of the situation, and it does not matter as much as it did. At first this may feel a little uncomfortable, but gentle perseverance will usually bring rewards.

2. REINFORCING FORMULA

This type is used to promote a change in a physiological response or a behavioural pattern.

Examples

If a student has natural apprehension about exams and is functioning well in their revision, an appropriate formula might be:

- *All my knowledge I recall,*
  In my exam I know it all.

If a child is bed-wetting, the recommended textbook formula is *'I know I wake up when my bladder is prompting'* (Luthe). For a child, this is somewhat bewildering. JB gave the following to the mother of a seven-year-old child who was wetting the bed at least five times per week:

- *I can wake to wee.*

The mother sat beside the child as she was going to sleep, gently repeating the phrase and encouraging her to take on the phrase as her last thought before sleep. Six weeks later, the report was one accident only. And that was because the child had been to a party and later said, 'I was too tired to use my sentence, Mummy'. She had readily accepted responsibility for her problem once she had found the solution for it. We should acknowledge here that the mother was using AT — it certainly helped her with the principle of standing back in dealing with the problem.

3. ABSTINENCE FORMULA
This type is used to break a habit or an addiction.

Examples

- *Smoking gives me up.*
- *Others may drink; for me alcohol does not matter.*
- *Cream doughnuts are not for me.*

The brain can stand back, be more detached about the issue.

4. PARADOXICAL FORMULA
Sometimes the direct opposite to the problem is used in a personal formula. This applies when extreme anxiety is present, and the balance can be corrected by the 'pendulum principle'. If the pendulum is stuck in an extreme pattern of behaviour, with attendant negative feelings (usually of anxiety), it may need a provocative route to release it so that it will swing to the opposite extreme. Now that it is moving, it will find its own balance with a new pattern. The paradoxical formula will act as that provocation.

Examples

- *I like to be messy* (for obsessive concern with housework).
- *I write as poorly as I can* (for writers' cramp).

This is appropriate only for those whose anxiety is not too great to use it. Telling the unconscious to go to the extreme opposite may increase the problem. You are the person to judge this — how does this form of wording you have chosen make you feel? If the answer is revulsion, increased fear or you simply forget to use it, move away from this type of approach.

5. SUPPORTING FORMULA

This approach gives a strong positive message to the brain that certain attitudes or behaviours are not only desirable but possible.

Example

- *I am sincere and trusting* (for improving a relationship).

This is probably the most commonly used type. Ensure that it is always in the present tense. But even here, be sure to check it out — is 'sincere' really the word you need here? If *you* interpret 'sincere' as suspect, associating it with its opposite — a 'sincere' smile could be put on, for example — then you may prefer to use 'genuine' instead. To you, 'genuine' may be less open for mis-interpretation than 'sincere'. So use the best word for you.

We are encouraging you to think carefully about all of this. A book can seem to have all the answers. Not so. What we present here are only ideas. You need to make them work in your style and your life.

> In Prague, on August 21st 1968, a Professor of Psychology was driving a visiting German professor though the city to the venue where he was due to lecture on Autogenic Therapy. The discussion naturally was about the merits of AT and the use of personal formulae. Suddenly they turned a corner and came face to face with a row of Russian tanks. The host professor froze, white-faced and sweating with fear. He then became aware of the voice of his passenger: 'Russian tanks leave me cool. Russian tanks leave me cool. Russian tanks ….'

> From Newsletter no. 27, July 1995.
> British Association for Autogenic Therapy and Training.

EXAMPLES OF PERSONAL FORMULAE OR AFFIRMATIONS

These are ideas only — for you to play around with perhaps the help of your therapist. Your own words are always best. You can start your phrases with any of the following:

- *I go with …*
- *I permit …*
- *I feel …*
- *I am …*
- *I allow …*
- *My ….*

Or you can use the principle of the passive automatic response:

- **It** *sleeps me.*

HEALTH MAINTENANCE

- *I heal myself.*
- *I listen to my body.*
- *My mind and body are as one.*
- *My internal vibrations are healthy.*
- *Healthy vibrations flow through my body.*
- *It heals me* (the immune defence system).
- *Smoking is giving me up.*
- *I care for my body/health.*

ACCEPTANCE OF SELF

- *I accept all my feelings as part of me.*
- *I love and respect myself.*
- *I acknowledge and accept myself completely.*
- *I am content with myself as I am.*
- *I am whole and complete in myself.*
- *I am worthy as I am.*

- *I release my entire past.*
- *I forgive and release myself.*
- *I am free.*
- *I have the right to be my true self.*
- *I am aware of my inner self, without conflict.*
- *My life is an adventure.*

MAINTENANCE OF WELL-BEING

- *Life and laughter are beautiful.*
- *I am well ordered and tranquil.*
- *I am filled with light and love.*
- *My crisis enables growth.*
- *I love to love and be loved.*
- *I am in charge of myself.*
- *I am calm, confident and assertive.*
- *I am calm and centred.*
- *I have plenty of time for everything.*
- *I am full of vitality.*
- *Laughter is happiness.*
- *I am happy enjoying myself.*
- *I am at peace with myself.*
- *Life is enjoyable.*
- *My world is beautiful.*
- *I am free of conflict.*
- *I release my guilt.*
- *I let go of my tension.*
- *I lecture with ease and confidence.*
- *Public speaking is fun.*
- *Audiences don't matter.*
- *I project warmth and understanding.*
- *People are fun to be with.*
- *Crowds don't matter.*
- *I sleep at night, calm and light.*
- *I sleep in the night without a fight.*

- *I wake up at 3, calm and free.*
- *I wake up at 5, calm and alive.*
- *I wake up at 7, calm and in heaven*
- *Waking doesn't matter* (sleep disturbance).
- *I easily wake up* (if waking is a problem).
- *Time does not matter* (overly time conscious).
- *Deadlines don't matter.*
- *Details don't matter* (obsessive tendency regarding details).
- *I let go of it.*
- *I enjoy my life despite the strife.*
- *Nobody is perfect* (perfectionism).
- *Winning is unimportant.*
- *Defeat does not matter.*
- *My voice does not matter.*
- *My mind is open to all that is spoken.*
- *It talks me.*
- *Dirt does not matter* (obsessive cleaning).
- *I want to be messy* (obsessive tidiness).
- *Comfort sleeps me* (insomnia*).*
- *My periods are calm and easy* (PMT).
- *It is calm and easy* (PMT).

MAINTENANCE OF REALITY

- *I am here now* (not in past or future).
- *I acknowledge my limitations.*
- *I acknowledge all that is me.*
- *I know myself.*
- *The world is incomplete without me.*
- *With my eyes I see all that is me.*
- *My ears are open to all that is spoken.*

MAINTENANCE OF RELATIONSHIPS

- *I forgive and release others.*
- *I am sincere and trusting.*

- *I accept and trust people.*
- *I attract loving attentions.*
- *I am orgasmic.*
- *I easily accept intimacy.*
- *I am loved and wanted.*
- *I release those I love.*
- *I trust those I love.*
- *I respect people.*
- *I love people.*
- *I love my neighbours as myself.*
- *I am receptive to people's needs.*
- *My love flows outwards.*
- *I project love and understanding.*
- *I project sensitivity.*
- *I open my heart to people.*
- *I am confident, receptive and flexible.*

FACILITATING CREATIVITY

- *My ideas are innovative.*
- *I am inventive.*
- *My mind is flexible.*
- *My mind shows me the way.*
- *Ideas flow from my mind.*
- *My ideas flow from my voice.*
- *My ideas flow through my fingers.*
- *My ideas flow through my pen.*
- *It flows with ideas* (the mind).
- *I open my mind to knowledge.*
- *I easily recall from memory.*
- *I easily retain information.*
- *I learn easily.*
- *Learning is fun.*
- *My voice is powerful.*
- *My voice is informative.*

- *My voice is influential.*
- *My voice is captivating.*
- *I am imaginative.*
- *My imagination is creative.*
- *I easily retain my studies.*
- *I recall everything easily.*

Never use the following words:

- *Must*   (implies pressure/striving)
- *Will*   (implies pressure/striving)
- *Ought*   (implies you might not)
- *Should*   (implies you might not)

Be aware of your feelings behind the change you wish to make. Rather than focus on '*panic goes away*' — build on the positive/opposite: '*I am confident and open*'; '*I am free to be myself*'.

Above all, **be gentle with yourself**.

PHYSICAL FORMULAE
(PREVIOUSLY KNOWN AS 'ORGAN-SPECIFIC FORMULAE')

These are specialised formulae which focus on bringing about a physical change. It is worth reminding ourselves that the system always looks after itself, and the Standard Exercise is the main tool for normal self-adjustment in the body. Time should be allowed for the process to do its work.

Later, you can build on your growing ability to observe and influence your body. You will begin to notice tensions earlier (before they manifest as pain) and take action to prevent them from developing.

These formulae have been misnamed in the past, as it is extremely unwise to experiment with formulae relating to the major organs. Always check with your therapist if you want to use a phrase relating to a specific organ.

Example

> Dr Luthe reported that a patient suffering from headaches decided that the opening formula about heaviness in her arm was not serving her needs, so she used 'My brain is heavy', thinking that it was more appropriate. Her headaches increased ten-fold, and it took Dr Luthe some time to dig out exactly what had gone wrong.

However, in a general context, some formulae affecting the physical condition are appropriate. Usually they enhance the effect of the Standard Exercise and are placed alongside the most appropriate standard formula.

For example, for poor circulation in the feet, after heaviness and warmth in the limbs, use '*My feet are (very) warm*'.

It is impossible to give a comprehensive list, although some suggestions follow.

SKIN

Itching
Often a formula suggesting coolness is good for itching.

- *My right hand is cool* (for a rash on the right hand — place after the phrase relating to arms and legs).
- *My eyes are cool* (for hay-fever — place after the forehead formula).

Most itching (such as is found in eczema) can be linked to a manifestation of anger. Skin is 'irritated' and we can feel frustrated and angered by the discomfort. Using 'cool and calm' directed to the affected part and placed appropriately in the Standard Exercise, is helpful, alongside Intentional Verbalisation of Anger Exercises.

ACUTE PAIN

Warmth or coolness is applied. Discuss with your therapist which is best. A good guide is to ask yourself whether you would normally apply a hot or cold pack for relief.

- *My right ankle is cool* (for a sprain. Place after the arms and legs phrase).

Arthritic pain may need a 'warm' approach:

- *My ankles/wrists are warm.*
- *My back is strong and supple.*

For a 'frozen' shoulder, or stiffness:

- *My* (right or left) *shoulder is warm.*

Other formulae would focus on breaking the cycle of pain:

- *I allow the (my) pain to float/seep/drift/wash away.*
- *I free myself from pain.*

CHRONIC PAIN

Discussion of pain often leads to generalised observations about its origins, which show up in our common language — 'Pain in the neck' (aggression, irritation), 'Carrying a lot on his shoulders' (burdens).

AT is very good at isolating pain to a specific area — by reducing or limiting the surrounding tension, which has been 'guarding' the pain. You can often reduce pain by 'making friends with it'. Then you may find that you can accept the pain better, watch and observe it, sometimes have a dialogue with the pain ('What are you saying to me?' 'What do you (pain) represent to me?' 'Do I really need you?')

Depending on the nature of the pain, a formula such as one of the following, can help:

- *Pain is unimportant — I feel comfortable.*
- *I allow myself to work through pain.*
- *I have no need of pain.*
- *There is no space/room in my life for pain.*
- *I free myself from pain.*
- *I am strong, healthy and pain-free.*

These can reduce the preoccupation with chronic pain.

Remember that some aches and pains are an indication for the use of Intentional Exercises. Pain is sometimes present because the person hasn't cried, or expressed anger and frustration, for a long time. The pain might increase to the extent that the person says, 'It's so bad I could cry.' When asked if they have cried, the reply will often be, 'Oh no I never let it get me down', or a shamefaced, 'Well — a bit'. This is a strong indicator of the need to use the Intentional Crying Exercise.

For example, chest pain and skin irritations may benefit from use of Intentional Verbalisation of Aggression, while itchy eyes and hay-fever, frontal headaches and sinusitis/catarrh need the Intentional Crying Exercise.

BOWEL AND DIGESTIVE PROBLEMS

The following may be added after the abdominal warmth exercise:

- *My lower abdomen is warm.*

Or you might focus on self-regulation:

- *My bowels function/empty normally.*

HAEMORRHOIDS (PILES)

- *My anus (arse? bum?) is heavy/cool. (Your own words are important.)*

BLADDER PROBLEMS

- *My bladder is warm and comfortable.*

COUGHING OR ASTHMA

- *My throat is cool, my chest is warm.*

FACIAL NEURALGIA

- *My jaw is heavy.*

All these formulae are used only for as long as they are needed — often very briefly. In some illnesses a more complicated formula may be used to encourage healing or normal functioning. Such a formula requires you to have a greater knowledge and understanding of the appropriate physiology, and you will need the help of your therapist to formulate it.

CAUTION

Be careful when you experience new symptoms. If they do not respond to autogenic techniques after a short time, they should be investigated.

CHAPTER 7

WHY WE NEED AUTOGENIC THERAPY

It is time to consider the reasons why we need AT to help us to gain optimum health. Much ill-health is influenced by lifestyle — perhaps we need to examine and change our behaviour in order to improve our health.

THE HOLISTIC APPROACH TO WELL-BEING

For many years, the conventional approach to good health has focused on the reduction or elimination of symptoms. Where possible, a cause for symptoms will be found, and also treated. But chronic symptoms, for which no cause comes to light, may linger for years, and bring about serious debilitation over time. These days, conventional medicine recognises the need for a holistic approach to health care, but the financial constraints of health services mean that provision of services still focuses on intervention only when things have gone wrong. Limited time and resources mean that the focus of treatment is often on reducing and managing symptoms, rather than treating the cause. While health education is supposedly aimed at the prevention of illness, we are still operating a reductionist method of keeping well. We have all been brought up to take 'our symptoms' to the doctor, rather than taking 'our whole selves'.

Costly technological advances and a growing population mean that things are unlikely to change in the near future. Medical training pays woefully little attention to the remarkable self-healing properties of the mind and body.

So, responsibility for good health rests more and more with the individual — a fact borne out in recent years by the increased use of complementary therapies.

STRESS

Many symptoms are now recognised as being stress-related, and the word is probably somewhat over-used. In our experience, the most common reason why people enquire about learning AT is that they are suffering from symptoms such as sleep disturbance, headaches, skin problems, fatigue, frustration, anxiety. All of these can be a reaction to too much stress.

The word 'stress' is often used as if to describe a complaint: 'I'm suffering from stress', 'My doctor says it's stress' — and yet 'stress' is not, in itself, a diagnosed illness. Stress becomes a problem only when we suffer an overload of it (di-stress).

There is nothing wrong with 'stress'. Historically, stress has stood us in very good stead, taking care of us by producing the 'stress' hormones adrenaline and noradrenaline when we are in danger. This sense of danger was, and still is, essential to our survival. We needed the adrenaline surge to prepare us instantly for flight or fight when we were under threat. These same hormones are also present when we are excited — perhaps anticipating a pleasurable event.

ONE MAN'S STRESS IS ANOTHER MAN'S PLEASURE
The glee with which scary rides at theme parks are undertaken illustrates the fine line between danger and excitement. Stress affects people in different ways. Some people actively seek out stressful activities — jumping from aeroplanes, climbing mountains, sailing solo, bungee jumping. We are all individual in our personality and physiological make-up, so there can never be a definitive prescription for the amount of pressure a person can take before they suffer ill effects. We cannot eliminate stress from our lives; we cannot necessarily change what is going on around us. But we *can* change how we react.

It is the way we react to stress — how we deal with it — that is the key. If we become aware that we constantly seem to be in a state of anxiety, high tension and frustration, perhaps we need to do something about it. So we are looking at 'stress' not as being a sole cause, but as being a catalyst or vehicle for unease, even illness.

Upbringing, life events and personality play their part, of course. When we are in good health and emotional balance, we are better able to take on new challenges, face events and cope with what life has to offer.

GOOD STRESS

In short manageable bursts, stress is good for us. We can rise to the challenge of a new job or project. And we can feel great satisfaction when that project is pushed to completion. We may have lost some sleep over it, but we can see the light at the end of the tunnel.

Dr Hans Selye's 1960s diagram showing the human organism's adaptability to stress, has been further developed here.

Without any stress or work pressure, there is no productivity. A continuum of unremitting and constant stress with no intervention leads to very serious problems.

Figure 8: Selye's Curve of Productivity (adapted)

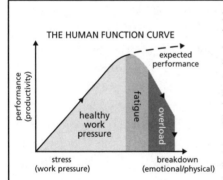

THE HUMAN FUNCTION CURVE

Healthy work pressure — you respond to the challenge of work pressure with enthusiasm, high energy and enjoyment, while maintaining a good balance in life outside work. Physical and mental health is good.

Fatigue — in this 'grey area', stress is increasing, fatigue sets in, and you push yourself harder. You neglect home and leisure, perhaps drinking too much alcohol, or suffering insomnia and minor complaints. There is mental frustration that your level of performance is ever harder to achieve. *This is the time to take positive steps to prevent serious problems.*

Overload — unremitting and constant stress can lead to feelings of being overwhelmed and isolated, and to loss of self-esteem and confidence. Physical symptoms worsen and, if left untreated, these feelings can lead to emotional breakdown (at worst, suicide) or physical breakdown (for example, heart attack).

If we learn to use Autogenic Therapy and literally re-educate the mind and body to respond differently to stress, we are putting ourselves into the best possible framework for dealing with it. We are also learning about ourselves. As we raise awareness about our personality and our limitations, and increase our sense of self-worth and confidence, we are better able to feel in control of our daily lives.

Defining Stress

In its book, *Managing Stress* (series No. 18, 'Managing Best Practice'), the Industrial Society defines stress thus:

> In this report 'stress' refers to negative changes in personal behaviour which result from an imbalance between pressure and people's current ability to cope with it.

This may not go far enough. In engineering terms, 'stress' is described as an external force applied to a rigid object. If this force is applied repeatedly, the object will retain its rigidity as far as possible, resisting the pressure. Eventually it will bend and distort its shape, until it breaks.

Imagine the same force applied to an elastic band: it is much more forgiving (adaptable), bouncing back time and again. The human being also bounces back, and adapts to pressure — it is one of the great gifts we have. We tend not to give in — we keep going, sometimes against all odds. How often do you find yourself shaking your head at the plight of others, saying, 'I don't know how they carry on. What must it be like, coping with all that?'

But we all know that eventually something will give. Symptoms will appear, or the person will have some kind of breakdown in physical or mental health (or social behaviour). Any of these indicate that the mind or body has had enough. Eventually there will be physical, emotional or social repercussions. The positive aspect of such events is that we have to stop, take time out and recover. We might feel terrible, but at the same time, it is *because* we are only human, and not machines, that we *can* react — hopefully in time for recovery to take place.

Example

Sheila had been widowed suddenly after a long marriage. The shock and sorrow were so great that for the first few months she had functioned 'on automatic pilot'. She stifled any emotion, always putting on a brave face and coping well. Then she began to drive herself on in life — taking up new activities, renewing old acquaintances, travelling. Two years after her husband's death, she began to suffer insomnia. Her doctor pre-scribed sleeping pills, which she refused every night, so she would often lie awake. As her energy decreased, she often felt 'unwell'. Her doctor told her that this was 'anxiety'. The insomnia and anxiety led her eventually to learn AT. Quite soon into the course, she had a few crying spells, and realised that she had never grieved properly. Her body had tried to tell her to take care. The symptoms were the warning. And eventually she heeded the warning. She allowed herself to be herself.

---

1. When Perceived Demand Exceeds the Resource to Meet it

You may feel that you have no control over a stressful job, or that you are trapped in situations you have no power to change. Pressures of work feel too much — there is simply too much to do and not enough time to do it. You react with symptoms such as insomnia, anxiety and some 'stress-related symptoms' such as Irritable Bowel Syndrome, skin problems or headaches. This kind of stress is about the present.

Today's lifestyle can be unrelenting. Recent research confirms that the UK is ahead of the rest of Europe in terms of stress at work, with long hours and pressure to out-perform competitors. The work ethic is linked with individual character traits such as perfectionism, or feeling not good enough. Office politics and fierce competition mean that job satisfaction is low, the next dead-line immediately follows the last, communications are so fast that there is no respite between projects. It is no longer possible to clear your desk at the end of the day. Your work follows you home — you find yourself receiving faxes at 2 a.m.

We spend most of our waking time in left-brain active concentration (see Chapter 2). We perceive the world around us as a constant stream of potential threats:

- Driving to work
- Dealing with aggressive people
- Listening to bad news stories
- Worrying about financial issues
- Feeling overburdened at work
- Feeling threatened by crime
- Fearing bereavement
- Caring for others (relationships)
- Worrying about accidents
- Worrying about illness.

So, if the stress is perceived as overwhelming, it becomes unbearable, converting itself to 'distress' (see Figure 8).

2. Stress as the Reaction of Mind and Body to CHANGE
Our lives are full of change. Take the initial arrival into the world at birth — the change from the warm, dark, safe womb to the bright, noisy bewildering outside world is terrifying, especially as it was preceded by our cosy world (womb) turning hostile and throwing us into the extraordinary journey. We can all remember times (quite normal in hindsight) when the new steps in our life journey have engendered strong emotions of doubt, loss, frustration and insecurity: the first day at school, changing schools, facing exams, leaving home, the first job, setting up home with a life-partner (add a wedding to the equation and you probably double the stress!) Each of these steps requires an adjustment of some kind in order to cope, as part of moving on to better things.

The key to surviving difficult life-changes is how we adapt to them. We have probably set up patterns of behaviour and attitudes which govern our reactions. It is possible to change the way the stressors in our lives affect us. We can change how we respond, and reduce our stress levels. Those who are prepared to accept responsibility for their actions and lifestyle can learn to regain control.

3. Stress as a Threat to Survival

Our physiology is designed to help us to cope with danger — the mouth goes dry, the heart pounds, fast; breathing turns to panting to increase oxygen to the blood supply to fuel the muscles which tense in readiness for '**fight**' (attack and slay the enemy) or '**flight**' (run away to safety). '**Fright**' or '**freeze**' is the third option, when you become paralysed and feel helpless — powerless to do anything to help yourself (likely to be the feeling in your worst nightmare).

These effects are the direct result of adrenaline (stress hormone) secretion.

All these responses from the secretion of adrenaline are a sure sign that our body is looking after us — very efficiently. And we instinctively know that these effects are a sign that we are in danger. Our panic is a safety mechanism, helping us to prepare for survival. We register the fear as though it were a real physical threat — it could equate to a feeling that there is a lion in the office! Our age-old safety mechanisms have been triggered by different stimuli. When we are rushed to get that report finished, when we are afraid that the boss will arrive and criticise us, we register the fear as though there really were a lion in the office. Our modern-day anxieties *are* related to survival after all. We're not going to be slain or eaten alive, but we perceive danger in the possibility that we might lose our jobs, be unable to pay the mortgage / support the family / keep our status.

The human organism is supremely sophisticated and finely tuned — it quickly adapts itself when in danger. Indeed, if our fight and flight mechanism *hadn't* been so efficient in our evolution, the human race would by now be extinct. But in today's world the problem lies in our inability to redress the balance. The danger signals get trapped inside us. Where do we put all that aggression and anxiety which the hormones have released? Some people 'take it out on the kids, the cat or the wife'. Others sensibly thrash balls around on a squash court, or use exercise to release pent-up aggression. Others abuse alcohol or substances. If we would only give ourselves the chance to rest, recuperate, recover and restore, as our ancestors did, we would allow our biological and emotional systems a chance to regain a state of equilibrium. Instead, we lurch from crisis to crisis, longing for the next holiday. But even then, it takes such a lot of organising (stress) to get away, and then we have to cope with the loss of routine, while spending every minute with other people. After the holiday, there's the prospect of returning to the office and 468 e-mails.

It's when we feel like this, and yet there is no lion, and we *know* that there is no lion, that we are in trouble. We may realise that we are often (perhaps constantly) in a state of underlying, non-specific anxiety or irritation. Or we have symptoms which we know increase when stress is around. The body can be in an almost constant state of fight or flight until the short-term benefits of the stress response become long-term problems (see Figure 9).

AT and the Reduction of Stress-Related Symptoms

When we practise an autogenic exercise, we feel at rest, at peace, in a pleasurable 'no-thought' state of mind. This is often described as the autogenic state, and it has a profound effect on the physiology of the mind and body.

Entering the autogenic state brings about a reversal of the stress response (see Figure 9), as governed by the sympathetic branch of the autonomic nervous system. During an autogenic exercise, many signs that this is the case can be noted: decreased muscle tension; reduced heart rate and breathing; general abdominal 'rumbles' indicating increased functioning of the abdominal organs. Over time, the immune system seems to get stronger (less prone to colds and infections); if measured, the blood pressure is shown to drop.

All this would imply that overall restoration of physiological functioning is taking place, as a direct result of the exercise.

Figure 9 shows how the physiological response initially kicks in to take care of us, what happens if it is too prolonged, and how AT can reverse it.

Figure 9: The 'Fight/Flight/Freeze' Response

THE BODY'S SPECIFIC RESPONSE TO STRESS THE 'FIGHT/FLIGHT/FREEZE' RESPONSE

Biological Response	Natural Short-Term Benefit	Long-Term Disadvantages if Unrelieved	Benefits of Autogenic Therapy
Release of cortisol from the adrenal glands	Protection from allergic reaction, asthma. Closing eyes from dust	*Weakens immune response. Impairs ability to fight disease*	*Strengthens immune response – less vulnerable to disease*
Adrenalin increases in the blood	Speeds up metabolism to provide extra energy	Anxiety, insomnia, exhaustion	Relief of anxiety. Improved sleep and energy
Release of endorphins	Pain killer	*Depleted levels aggravates migraines and other aches and pains*	*Restores body's ability to cope with pain*
Digestive tract shuts down	Blood diverted to heart, lungs, muscles and brain, ready for action	Dry mouth, bloating, nausea, cramps, diarrhoea and constipation	Restores normal working of the gut
Release of sugar and insulin into the blood	*Quick short distance energy for flight or fight*	*Blood sugar fluctuates. Diabetes aggravated*	*Blood sugar more evenly balanced*
Increase in cholesterol	Takes over energy supply when sugar runs out	Increased cholesterol in the blood	Evidence of long-term cholesterol reduction
Increased heart rate	*To carry oxygen and fuel*	*Raised blood pressure can lead to stroke or heart attack*	*Evidence shows possible long-term reduction in blood pressure*
Increased breathing rate	Provides extra oxygen	Hyperventilation and respiratory problems	Restores normal breathing patterns
The blood thickens	*Increases capacity to carry oxygen, fight infection and reduce bleeding*	*Increased risk of stroke, heart attack and clots*	*Reduces cardiac risk factors*
Skin crawls, pales and sweats	Blood goes to vital organs	Circulation problems. Cold extremities	Restores normal resting circulation
Senses become acute	*Brings the body to its peak of function. Improves mental function*	*Senses become less efficient: poor concentration and decision making*	*Increased self-awareness: concentration, clarity, alertness*

Figure 10 shows many symptoms or behaviour patterns which are signals that all is not well. When these are experienced as 'long-term' or 'chronic', the person needs help to alleviate the stress response.

Figure 10: Symptoms Related to Stress Excess (di-stress)

Sleep Problems
Inability to switch off in order to get to sleep; frequent waking through the night; waking up early with the mind racing; need to sleep all the time; constant fatigue.

Anxiety
Constant worry for no reason; fretting about unimportant things; racing heart; breathing problems; imagining the worst; guilt feelings; avoidance of stressful activities; sweating; blushing; panic attacks; worsening phobias.

Irritability/Impatience
Annoyance over trivial things; snapping at people; short temper; hatred of waiting or queuing; aggression; blaming others; constant dislike of things and people; feelings of resentment.

Physical Problems
Headaches; migraine; muscular tension leading to aches and pains; increased infections; neck problems; lower back pain; digestive problems; worsening allergies; hyperventilation ('over-breathing'); hypertension (high blood pressure); poor sports performance.

Psychological Problems
Loss of interest; depression; social withdrawal; feelings of insecurity; feelings of rejection.

Poor Mental Functioning
Lack of concentration (headless chicken mode); poor memory; inability to make decisions; diminishing creativity; inability to prioritise.

Increased Mannerisms
Nail-biting, finger-picking; fiddling with hair or face; biting of lips or inside the mouth; coughing; swallowing; blinking; drumming of fingers; incessant talking.

Increased Use of Unhealthy Substances
High caffeine intake; excessive smoking; excessive drinking of alcohol; excessive use of self-medication; use of illegal drugs.

Eating Problems
Eating junk food; craving too many sweet foods, causing blood-sugar swings; eating too much; eating too little.

Anti-Social Behaviour
Law-breaking; promiscuity; destructive behaviour.

STRESS-RELATED CAUSES OF PREMATURE DEATH

The six commonest causes of death under the age of 65 years can all be linked with a stressful lifestyle:

- Cardiovascular disease
- Cancer
- Accidents
- Pneumonia and influenza
- Cirrhosis of the liver
- Suicide.

SELF-RIGHTING MECHANISMS

The human organism takes care of itself, as we have seen above. Bones mend, tissue heals, infection is fought — all naturally. The mind and the body are sensitive to the prevailing internal and external conditions, and constant adjustments are made to maintain our physiological and emotional well-being.

So, it stands to reason that even when we feel bad ('stressed out'), the signal is there for us to respond to, if we choose. We may take some time to find the right path, but we should listen and respond to these inherent signals.

There is a name for this self-righting mechanism:

> HOMEOSTASIS The tendency towards a relatively stable equilibrium between interdependent elements, especially as maintained by physiological processes.
>
> (Oxford English Dictionary)

Botanists know this, as part of the study of plants. Homeostasis is equally applicable to the human organism. Dr Luthe's definition is:

> The perfect functional harmony of all the physiological and biochemical processes in mind and body.

So astonishing is the design of the human organism (brilliant, complex and unbelievably sophisticated) that often we do not heed it. If we imagine ourselves back to the moment of conception — when the sperm and egg first merged — it is likely that there was very little wrong at that time. The two cells functioned and multiplied in harmony with each other. As long as the environment remains optimal for all the correct processes to take place, the likelihood of 'functional imbalance' is minimal. In other words, left to its own devices, the human being is well balanced and self-righting.

This is the human organism — constantly in a state of adaptation, readjustment, and rebalancing of itself, striving for homeostasis. So when it throws up symptoms which persist, we need to listen to them. Your body knows best — it will always tell you when it's in trouble. But do you know how to listen to it? Have you ignored it for so long that it needs to produce a pain to claim your attention? That's where learning AT can help, teaching you to become the expert on yourself.

'DOING' VERSUS 'BEING'

Our culture does not encourage the sort of activity that allows recovery. If we daydreamed as a child (naturally tapping into our self-righting processes), this was frowned upon and we were punished. As adults, we perceive 'doing nothing' as a sin — we are encouraged to be constantly striving for results, always occupied in 'useful' pursuits — so we feel guilty if we do nothing. This shows that we have forgotten how to 'be'. We need to be able to switch to a passive neutral state, with regular frequency.

Emotional responses are suppressed for social reasons, and this can also inhibit natural recuperation processes. Our activities, attitudes and beliefs are a major influence on that balance. It is worth looking at our behaviour in terms of whether it is working towards our good balance (pro-homeostatic) or against it (anti-homeostatic).

ANTI-HOMEOSTATIC BEHAVIOUR (AGAINST HOMEOSTASIS)

We often indulge in anti-homeostatic behaviour because periods of stress affect our motivation to follow healthy activities. These types of behaviour can be presented in various categories.

Physical

- *Poor diet.* It often seems as if there is no time or energy to spend on ourselves, so we go for the easy options — such as eating junk food — which cause fluctuating blood-sugar levels. Continuing these erratic eating habits leads to many health problems.
- *Lack of exercise; excessive exercise.* We may give up our regular exercise, although sometimes there can be an obsession to exercise, and an addiction to the endorphins released. The latter requires greater and greater levels of exercise to give gratification.
- *Exposure to chemicals; drug abuse; smoking.* Under stress, we may turn to chemical substances, alcohol, caffeine, nicotine, self-medication or illegal substances in an attempt to gain short-term relief.
- *Exposure to disease; dangerous sport; rest deprivation.* We may expose ourselves to accidents by indulging in activities such as reckless driving or risk-taking in dangerous sport. We may stay up late, in order to 'fit more in', or wake early and start again.

Emotional

- *Aggressive, impatient or obsessive behaviour.* This not only affects those around us, damaging relationships, but has strong links with heart disease.

- *Suppression of emotion; negative imagination.* These can lead to a variety of problems (see Chapter 5). Worrying about things beyond our control or imagining bad things happening can have a destructive effect.
- *Boredom; lack of mental stimulation.* Lack of gratification, under-achieving — these can lead to depression.

Social

- *Isolation.* We often withdraw from social activity during busy times. This leaves us detached, without the benefit of support from others, or the sharing of common feelings that give us a sense of belonging and community in the world.
- *Debt; law-breaking.* These can lead to high levels of anxiety. We might spend money for comfort (retail therapy).
- *Wrong job.* Being in the wrong job or relationship means that our true potential cannot be fulfilled, and this leads to frustration.
- *Promiscuity.* We could be at risk from sexually transmitted disease from ill-considered sexual encounters, which may be sought out for some sort of immediate gratification. This can also result in feelings of guilt, and may destroy supportive relationships.
- *Excessive change.* If we are exposed to constant life-changes (good or bad), we need time to adapt, but when we are functioning under pressure we ignore this need.
- *Excessive competitiveness.* This leads to stress and social isolation.
- *Exposure to negative media images.* We are bombarded with repetitive graphic representation of horrific world events over which we have no control. This can lead to raised anxiety levels.

PRO-HOMEOSTATIC BEHAVIOUR (TOWARDS HOMEOSTASIS)
In order to help the system to stay in balance, our behaviour needs to satisfy physical, emotional, social, and spiritual needs. More positive behaviour patterns will directly influence our well-being.

Why We Need AT

Physical

- *Healthy diet.* We know that what we eat plays a great part in our health and well-being. Some foods have very positive effects on physical well-being. It is important to be aware that what you eat is contributing to physical growth and repair, and to the way you look and feel.
- *Exercise.* Exercise encourages systems of the body to work efficiently. Making muscles and joints work keeps them in good condition. This includes the muscles of the heart and lungs. Exercise also produces hormones that lift the mood and make us feel good. It also plays a part in maintaining our optimum weight.
- *Sleep.* Sleep is needed to help us to recuperate from the activities of the day. Both physical recuperation and emotional recuperation go on while we sleep. (See Chapter 9.)
- *Laughter.* Laughter is very healthy, both physically and emotionally, and keeps our immune systems in a good state of balance. Laughter helps circulation and lung efficiency and produces hormones that make us feel good.
- *Sex.* Sexual activity, if performed as part of a loving relationship, also helps to keep us in good working order.
- *Rest and recreation.* Diversion from our normal daily activity allows for recuperation of all the physiological systems.

Emotional

- *Love.* It is very important to have in our lives people whom we care for and trust — those whom we feel we can be ourselves with, can talk to about our joys and sorrows, people who will stand by us and give us support, no matter what.
- *Praise.* When we receive from others and from ourselves acknowledgement for achievements, it gives us a sense of our own worth. (Sometimes it is an achievement to get out of bed in the morning.)

- *Time and space for self.* Time and space for reflection, to consider where we are going, are very necessary for our well-being, helping us to make good life choices.
- *Mental activity.* As we progress through life, we learn new skills and gain from our experiences. Without this, we can become bored and depressed.
- *Control of own life.* If we feel that we do not have any control over what is happening to us, and we are unable to make our own decisions about our lives, we could become depressed and give up trying to look after our own welfare.
- *Positive outlook.* Looking optimistically at the world helps us to feel good and to make positive decisions.
- *Self-esteem.* The better our opinions of ourselves, the more care we will give to ourselves.
- *Confidence.* We cannot take risks, in order to improve our lives, without a degree of confidence. We need to be able to experiment, to find new ways of developing ourselves and to make positive decisions. A strong sense of 'self' (ego) helps our personal growth.
- *Expression of emotions.* We know that excessive 'bottling up' of emotions leads to many different physical and emotional problems. Once we accept our emotions as a part of who we are, we can learn to express them appropriately, and realise that they play an important part in keeping us healthy.

Social

- *Companionship.* Being around other people, listening to what is going on in their lives, and being able to share experiences, gives us a good sense of how we're doing in the world, and keeps things in proportion.
- *Mentor/confidant(e):* A wise friend to talk to and reflect with us will help us to make the right choices in life, and keep a good life balance.
- *Hobbies.* These act as an escape route — a means of leaving our difficulties aside for a while. When we are absorbed in the

process of creating something, whether it be making bread or carving lumps of stone, we are put in touch with the rest/ recuperation side of our brains. Later we can face other problems with renewed energy.

- *Flexible attitudes.* In this modern world, we are constantly dealing with change. If we are unable to adapt to the changing attitudes, beliefs and behaviour around us, we find ourselves out of balance and in conflict.
- *Arts and nature.* Looking at beauty helps us to feel good, and gives us a sense of the world around us. Being close to nature, acknowledging and appreciating the changing seasons, gives us a sense of time and place in the universe, which is very balancing.
- *Holidays.* When we are free to do as we choose, and we can let go of the usual rules of life, our equilibrium is restored. (This is provided that you don't bump up your stress levels in the preparation for it!)

Spiritual

- *Belief system; freedom of religion.* Having a belief in things spiritual, whether from formalised religion or other individual philosophies and systems, gives us an added sense of ourselves in a wider perspective of being. It allows us to explore things outside the material world, beyond our present knowledge; it helps us to expand the potential of our minds and connect with a greater universal wisdom.

PSYCHOSOMATIC SYMPTOMS — THE MIND/BODY LINK

PSYCHOSOMATIC SYMPTOMS AND SOMATISATION

Here we must look at an interesting, and at times confusing, area. We have all heard of psychosomatic symptoms. A psychosomatic symptom does not have a physical origin, but springs from the mind causing a symptom which provides a question-mark about the presence of clinical disease. This is often interpreted as a disparaging explanation/diagnosis — *'My doctor told me I am imagining my symptoms', 'I'm told my symptoms are all in the mind — but they're not — I really do have pain'*. This often leaves us feeling that nothing can be done about it. But when we look again at the word 'psychosomatic', we find that there is truth behind it, and its meaning is not at all critical or dismissive. The word derives from the Greek *psyche*, meaning 'mind', and *soma* meaning 'body'. So, a symptom that is 'somatised' and does not show a pathological or clinical change in the body could very well have its origin in the mind. *Psychosomatic* means 'of the mind and body'.

This is very good news for us — there is plenty we can do about it. However, we need to encourage an open mind so that we are able to address any psychological implications as they arise. Sometimes people feel frightened to do this — they might associate a psychological issue with a psychiatric illness (which, in turn, they associate with going mad). Rather, it is more likely to be related to emotional issues which have not been resolved. When they discover that AT is well within their power to learn and use, and that it seems to do a job more powerful than they might have expected, true relief is experienced. (We have to say, this is the spark which gives autogenic therapists their huge job satisfaction.)

A multitude of symptoms could be psychosomatic. They range from headaches to unexplained abdominal pain; from muscle tension to chronic pain; from hormonal disturbance to chest pain. It is, of course, important to distinguish between organic illness and psychosomatic symptoms. Before taking them on for AT, every autogenic therapist will carefully question a prospective client to ensure that symptoms such as chest pain have been investigated for clinical cause.

Some psychosomatic symptoms may be the result of past trauma, the memory of which has been buried, not expressed or released. These memories can be triggered at any time. We have often observed how memories can resurface for clients who were traumatised in childhood, either around the time of the birth of their own children, or when the child reaches the same age as when their own trauma occurred.

The body takes on the negative effect of the buried memory, creating a genuine physical symptom. The original psychological denial may have stood us in good stead at the time — for example, attempting to protect us as children from pain which felt too big to deal with. That's what our defence systems are all about. The autogenic process will usually address these issues, and the prompt for doing so is the psychosomatic symptom which is not responding to conventional approaches.

The first step in dealing with any psychosomatic symptom is to accept it as normal. It is there, alerting you to the fact that attention is needed. As long as you fight it, or try to smother it (using drugs to 'kill it' perhaps), you will actually be encouraging it to stick around, because you are not acknowledging what it stands for. If you appreciate the part it is playing in your make-up, listening to the discomfort it is giving you, you will learn during your exercises to tolerate it; it will act as a barometer for you — measuring your progress through the AT course. And it is likely eventually to disappear altogether.

There is no doubt that the mind and the body operate as foils for each other. If the body is ill, the mind probably doesn't feel very well either. Sufferers of ME (or Chronic Fatigue Syndrome) often complain that some doctors believe that depression is the root of their symptoms. Their answer is to say, '*Wouldn't you feel depressed if you had ME — constant pain and exhaustion, month in and month out? Being forced to give up work and all the things which make up your life is not a conscious choice — of course I'm depressed.*'

We are often more susceptible to colds and general bugs when we feel low. A depressed person (mind) is likely to have a depressed immune system (body), and therefore is more prone to picking up infection.

Even our language and ways of speech lead us into the Mind–Body connection. Think of phrases we use every day, which relate to how we feel (emotions). Many of them relate to what's going on in the body:

- *So-and-so makes me sick* (usually an angry statement).
- *I need to get it off my chest* (a need to release feelings of anger, sadness, anxiety or fear?)
- *He's a pain in the neck / He gives me a pain* (he makes me angry).
- *What's eating you?* (stomach ulcer)
- A skin rash usually evokes anger: it *irritates*.

Summary
Feeling (stress/emotion) causes a *physiological response:* a psychosomatic (of mind and body) symptom.

Case 1 — Joanna
Joanna was 40, and had been using AT for several years. Then her life was hugely disrupted by the presence of builders in the family home — the chaos lasted for six months, and she coped with working at home, family demands and all the rest! Never having suffered from any form of skin problem before, she was surprised when a small patch of eczema developed on her right hand, between the thumb and index finger. The patch would increase in size and density, then subside again, but it refused to clear. Joanna then realised that this was her 'barometer' of stress. She accepted it with interest, following its progress as the weeks passed. She applied creams only occasionally. The week after the builders had finished, the patch cleared up, never to return. (The builders had frequently remarked how calm she was, putting up with all the mess. One said that it was the calmest house he had ever worked in. So her skin expressed the stress for her — psychosomatic indeed!)

EMOTIONAL RELEASE
In a deeply relaxed state, when all other distraction is removed, the mind will tap into any unresolved emotional issues in its attempt to restore equilibrium. This is an opportunity to work through

and resolve this material, on both a conscious and an unconscious level. If this material is not addressed, physical and emotional problems can result, inhibiting personal growth and development.

It is often such difficulties which prompt someone to learn AT.

Only he who lets himself be can be himself

Schultz

MOVE TOWARDS AUTHENTIC SELF

When emotional and physical health have been restored, and the habit of regular 'time out' for autogenic exercises is in place, the use of deep relaxation leads us to the next part of the process — personal growth and development.

We have found that many people report extra dimensions to their lives when they have learned AT. These may be:

RELEASE OF CREATIVITY
Example: One woman decided to buy a piano and fulfil a life-long dream by learning to play.

DEVELOPMENT OF A SPIRITUAL AWARENESS
Example: A committed Christian found that his ability and willingness to pray were greatly enhanced.

GREATER SELF-KNOWLEDGE, AWARENESS AND INSIGHT INTO OWN NEEDS
Example: A City banker moved to Norfolk to breed pigs.

GREATER UNDERSTANDING OF THE WORLD, AND TOLERANCE OF OTHERS
Example: An industrial manager transformed himself from being a tyrant to being a caring human being.

CONFIDENCE TO MOVE TOWARDS MEETING YOUR NEEDS
Example: A young woman with ME found that she was no longer afraid of her anger, was able to express it assertively, and pace herself better, avoiding tiredness.

Figure 11: A Summary of Why You Might Choose to Learn AT

Practising autogenic therapy means:

- *You are taking responsibility for yourself.*
  You are your own best therapist — with your new self-awareness.
  AT helps you towards renewed energy for making changes.
  You can change only yourself — not other people.

- *You are looking after your health.*
  Being physically fit helps to cope with stress.

- *You can learn to accept yourself.*
  Recognise your unique potential and move towards achieving it.

- *You can learn to recognise and appreciate your own achievements.*
  Be less reliant on the perceived opinions of others.

- *You can learn to take time for yourself.*
  Take holidays.
  Give yourself some time and space each day.
  Be at ease with doing nothing.

- *You can spend more time on relaxing enjoyable activities.*
  Read, listen to music.
  Be entertained.

- *You can find increased creative outlets.*
  Find new interests and hobbies
  Appreciate and become absorbed in the process of activities, rather than in the end product.

- *You can take more interest in the environment.*
  Seek out nature, spending more time in the fresh air.
  Exposure to daylight stimulates the production of serotonin and helps with mood and sleep.
  You may renew your own environment, clearing out clutter, redecorating.

- *You can learn to be at peace without feeling guilty.*
  Contemplate, meditate, be at ease with serenity.

- *You can learn to question your rules …*
  … especially those you impose on others. They may no longer be relevant.
  Imposing rules may lead to unnecessary arguments and stress.

- *You may be able to change your routine to make better use of your time.*
  Stop doing things from habit rather than necessity.

- *You may find new joy in your family, displaying your positive feelings more readily.*

- *You can improve your social life.*
  Be more confident in social situations.

- *You can retrieve your sense of humour.*
  Laughter is excellent stress relief.

- *You can learn to think positively.*
  Stop your negative imagination from running riot.

- *You can learn to ask for help*
  You are worthy of it.

- *Above all, you will learn to be kind to yourself.*

CHAPTER 8

APPLICATIONS OF
AUTOGENIC THERAPY

The potential areas of application of Autogenic Therapy are many and various. AT is *so* good, has *so* much potential in how it can change lives, that we are in constant danger of sounding like evangelical proponents of a miracle cure-all. It is not that AT itself is a cure — more that the potential for it to do good in many different areas should not be ignored.

In this and the following chapter, we will address many physical and psychological symptoms and conditions which AT has been known to help. We will look at some of the great variety of personal experiences that have come our way. In Chapter 9, we include areas and stories of performance: in the workplace, sport, theatre, dance, music, creativity.

People usually seek out AT because they have a problem. Often this problem is connected with their health — either physical or emotional. If they have sought advice, they have often drawn a blank in terms of a clinical answer, or treatment has had only a limited effect. Now they are looking for a new avenue — a complementary approach, or some form of stress management. Above all, they are looking for something they can do to help themselves, perhaps as an alternative to drugs. (*'Isn't there something I can do?' 'I want to do something myself.'*)

Where we had come to believe that the state and the health service would keep us healthy, we now realise that we have to take more responsibility for our own health. Those seeking AT are taking that responsibility.

As we explain a little about various conditions and symptoms which can be helped by AT, bear in mind that many symptoms overlap, or arise from one another. A psychological symptom can be a natural response to a physical one, and vice versa. We are not saying that AT is always the complete answer, nor is it within the remit of this book to list all the possible remedies for a given condition.

Some changes in lifestyle and/or some additional treatment are often necessary. In this respect, AT helps to raise awareness of what is needed, and to increase the motivation to change what you can. AT will also enhance the positive effects of other therapies. For example, a chiropractor will find you more receptive to their treatment; the dentist will appreciate the marked reduction in resistance.

Symptom improvement will obviously vary from person to person, depending on many factors, including their dedication to practising AT. In general, we do not follow up all our clients in the long term. Where long-term follow-ups have been done, changes brought about in the first four months of using AT (this period is taken from initial assessment to follow-up) have been shown to increase over time.

PSYCHOSOMATIC SYMPTOMS AND SOMATISATION

Psychosomatic symptoms and somatisation were discussed in Chapter 7.

In many of the cases that follow, you may detect an element of psychosomatic influence.

ARTHRITIS

Recent research has shown evidence of a positive benefit from AT for sufferers of arthritis, including improvement in their blood chemistry (see Chapter 12). AT can help with chronic pain, and relaxation of the muscles surrounding a swollen and painful joint will improve general comfort. Improved blood circulation (through the warmth exercise) helps to increase the efficiency of the body's own defences, and may reduce the reliance on medication. Using Intentional Exercises may well address some emotional issues which might have contributed to the condition.

Case 1 — Hannah

This woman, in her seventies, learned AT to help her chronic arthritis. Her domineering mother had lived with her and her husband all their married life, and 'ruled her with a rod of iron', eventually dying in her nineties. Hannah had had no opportunity for self-expression. She saw little of her daughter, not wishing to be domineering like her mother. Through using AT, her joints became freer, she gained relief from pain and improved her mobility. She also used the Intentional Exercises and found a great source of release with them. Her anxiety levels decreased and she was able to cope better with life in general.

BLADDER DISORDERS

Functional disorders in micturition (the ability to pass urine) may well have a strong psychological component, in which case the Standard Exercises contribute a lot to improvement. These symptoms have been known to be relieved by using the Intentional Crying Exercise. Benefits have been noted in the following circumstances:

- Frequency of urination
- Nocturnal enuresis (bed-wetting in children)
- Inability to pass urine in public toilets
- Post-operative urinary retention

Case 1 — Juliet

At 24, Juliet found life very restricting as, in any stressful situation, she had to empty her bladder at frequent intervals — at worst, this might have been every half hour. This meant organising life so that she was always within reach of a toilet. Following the AT course, her anxiety levels were generally much reduced, and if her bladder did prompt at awkward times, she used her personal formula — 'My bladder is warm and comfortable' — and she was able to override the urge.

CARDIOVASCULAR PROBLEMS

The best use of AT for this body system is as a preventive strategy.
Dr Brian O'Donovan writes:

> Autogenic Therapy cannot be expected to reverse perma-
> nent damage to the heart, vascular system or any other body
> system ....
>
> Treatment is of value: In prevention of serious heart dis-
> ease; as a valuable adjunct to the treatment of angina; to
> increase coronary blood flow and reduce (high) blood pres-
> sure; as non-specific psycho-physiologic relaxation; in the
> recovery phase after infarction (heart attack) and to prevent
> further attacks; to prevent the need for coronary-artery
> surgery or for rehabilitation after such surgery.
>
> Dr Brian O'Donovan, *AT in Organic Illness*

There is no doubt that using AT will help to prevent heart disease
by reducing cardiac risk factors. Research has shown that high and
borderline blood pressure has reduced, and high cholesterol levels
respond favourably to regular practice of Standard AT Exercises.
The latter shows that it may be the metabolism of cholesterol
which is more significant in reducing cholesterol levels than
dietary measures.

AT is also very helpful in the recovery process after hospitalisation for a heart attack. It should not be undertaken too soon
after the event, but your therapist will guide you.

OTHER RELATED AREAS WHERE AT CAN HELP

Angina
Here AT can be of great therapeutic value, especially in promot-
ing relaxation and a general letting go of anxiety associated with
the condition. Some clients manage to reduce their medication
for angina.

Case 1 — Sue

Sue, aged 50, with young adult children and a busy life teaching, was suddenly diagnosed with a type of angina (chest pain which occurs when relaxing, rather than the usual kind — on exertion. Having always regarded herself as fit, she had to cope with the shock of ill-health as well as invasive treatment. She surprised herself by how much she could reverse her fears by expressing them. She also found that she was at ease with her own emotions, and able to deal with them on her own, rather than resorting to over-analysis and 'attention-seeking' from her partner. Her heart condition may not alter in a physical sense, but Sue feels that she now has the control — the power to prevent things from getting any worse.

Chest Pain

Chest pain which has been investigated, and no abnormality found, often has a psychological background, such as the suppression of anger ('*I need to get it off my chest*'). Autogenic therapy is very helpful in reducing physical and psychological tension, allowing reduction of the symptoms and reassurance for the client.

Case 2 — Robin

Robin was in his fifties, with a job he was finding increasingly frustrating. When he felt under stress, he experienced worsening chest pains. Through his GP he underwent a series of routine tests, which revealed no physical cause for his pain. He was recommended AT for 'stress' and, although somewhat cynical, he agreed and carried out the tasks as instructed. Within a few weeks, he noticed reduction of pain. Robin was able to recognise the triggers and even ward off the pain. He felt more laid back in general, coping with stressful situations, and by the end of the course his chest pain was a thing of the past.

Circulation

By allowing a normalisation of blood flow to the peripheral vessels, AT can be helpful in a range of circulatory problems.

Case 3 — Sheila (chilblains)

A 44-year-old secretary, Sheila had suffered chilblains for most of her life. Whatever she did to try to prevent them, her toes swelled and itched every winter, causing much discomfort. She learned AT in the autumn, and reported no recurrence of chilblains five years later.

Case 4 — Annette (Raynaud's Disease)

Annette, aged 46, married with a growing family, had suffered from very painful fingertips for more than twenty years. In the coldest weather she would suffer infections which were not only very inconvenient (requiring constant attention with dressings), but also extremely painful. After a few weeks of using AT, her pain increased quite unexpectedly, since it was late May, then receded, and since then her fingers are a much-improved colour and pain-free.

Hypertension (high blood pressure)

This is understood to be one of the precipitating factors for possible heart attack or stroke, so concern is always present where there are consistently high readings. Blood pressure can vary according to circumstance, and a 'labile blood pressure' is one which seems to fall or climb according to the weather or the day of the week. Self-monitoring is usually a good way to reduce the anxiety surrounding readings, and avoids too much of the 'white-coat syndrome' which is associated with going to the doctor to 'have it taken'.

For some, AT is a great help in reducing high blood pressure. It is important to have your blood pressure monitored during a course, so if you are taking medication, do not stop until you are sure, from consultation with your doctor, that it is safe to do so. Sometimes a paradoxical rise in BP will show up during the AT course, but this usually settles again of its own accord.

Myocardial Infarction (heart attack)

If you have suffered a heart attack, you will already have been advised of the merits of using relaxation as part of your recovery programme. We would not advise an MI patient to learn AT until at least three — perhaps six — months after the event. The relaxation component of AT will be very beneficial of course, but AT has also helped the after-effects of health- (heart-) related anxiety. Sometimes a condition called 'cardiac neurosis' develops after a heart attack, where the patient develops quite severe anxieties around the issue of their heart, activities and energy levels. AT usually helps this to resolve, which in turn aids the recovery on an emotional basis as well the physical.

Case 5 — Peter (heart attack)

Peter was 63 when he learned AT, a year after he had been in hospital with a heart attack. His recovery had been uneventful, but he was left with some anxiety about the whole event. He found himself 'listening out' for his heartbeat a lot of the time. When he reached the exercise about cardiac regulation in his AT course, his therapist wondered if it might be better to leave it out for a few weeks, until he was further on with his process. As he was in a group, the new formula was introduced anyway, allowing him a chance to comment on it. His face lit up and he said, 'This one's for me — it's what I've been waiting for.' He found it reassuring and relaxing — as though 'all is well with me and my heart'.

CHRONIC PAIN

Some conditions leave people with a problem with chronic and unremitting pain. Management of this is important in order to improve the quality of life. It is useful to explore the psychological implications of such pain — such as anxiety and depression — and put the Intentional Off-loading Exercises to good use. Sometimes chronic pain leaves the client perceiving themselves as the victim of circumstance, with no control over their lives. This attitude might interfere with their progress with AT — letting go of the pain may mean that they have to face up to other issues. The use of personal formulae are of great help here (see Chapter 7).

Case 1 — Lisa

This 34-year-old had suffered from chronic shoulder and back pain for eight years, since a bad car accident. She had had several episodes of surgery, but was left with severe difficulties. During the AT course, she addressed her grief for the loss of her good health and pain-free life, and she addressed her anger about the crash and the people who had caused it. Using the Intentional Crying Exercise had brought much relief, as she had formed the habit of holding on to her feelings in order not to upset others, or 'be a nuisance'. She could also express her anxiety about her future with the Intentional Verbalisation of Anxiety Exercise — most of the work was about giving herself permission to be honest about her feelings. Amazingly, her pain got more controllable, and she began to make plans for her future.

DIGESTIVE (GASTRO-INTESTINAL) SYSTEM DISORDERS

CONSTIPATION

Even if the reason for learning AT has nothing to do with constipation, reports are often favourable. Tension, emotional upset, stress — all these can cause difficulties in the digestive system, even for those who normally eat a good diet. AT will often encourage the bowel quite spontaneously to return to a good evacuation habit. Introducing warmth to the area can add reinforcement if needed.

Luthe's colleagues conducted a study, using heaviness only, on sixteen patients who had suffered from constipation for more than two years. The use of laxatives was forbidden unless absolutely necessary, and monitoring continued over a two-year period. Four people dropped out, preferring the laxative method(!); two did not bring about any change in their symptoms; one improved his symptoms markedly, but stopped using AT. The remaining nine people were completely cured — six of these noticed that normal bowel habits began in the first two to three weeks of practising heaviness.

It is worth remembering that repressed anger is often a component of constipation. 'Holding in the rubbish' could be what is going on here — a good indicator for using the Intentional Verbalisation of Aggression Exercise.

CROHN'S DISEASE AND ULCERATIVE COLITIS

These conditions of inflammation of the small and large intestines respectively tend to respond well to AT, although perseverance is needed — a minimum of a few months' practice is usually required. Most autogenic therapists subscribe to the view that these unpleasant symptoms have their root in suppressed anger. The determination of the person is paramount here — coupled with a willingness to understand and accept the emotional component in their symptoms.

Case 1 — Janet

Janet, a 35-year-old civil servant and mother of three, suffered from Crohn's Disease (affecting the small bowel), which was her main reason for learning AT. At the start of the course, she had just weaned herself off a course of steroid drugs and was hoping to avoid having to take them again. Her usual pattern was that after a course of steroids a flare-up of her condition would occur within a few weeks, which would necessitate another course.

She had sometimes in the past complained of needing to sleep 'too much'. During her AT course, this increased to quite a worrying degree. At the weekend she would sleep for seventeen hours at a stretch. And yet she was able to keep going at work, and in her demanding home-life. (Her therapist was concerned that this might be a contraindication for AT — that Janet suffered from narcolepsy, falling asleep all the time, and in the most unlikely circumstances. However, Janet stayed awake in all the AT sessions, which was an indicator that all was well, so it was decided to monitor carefully without specific action.)

After six weeks, Janet reported that her sleep pattern had returned to normal, and that she now had much more energy. She felt that the fifth Standard Exercise had helped her a great deal — her Crohn's symptoms were 'quiet' and she hoped for a continued symptom-free period. She definitely felt that she was much more in control of her medical condition.

By the eighth week, Janet had stopped taking her regular medication for Crohn's, as her symptoms had improved so much. So far they had not recurred. She was aware that all the sleep was connected with her recovery process. She described the need as feeling as though it was compulsive — she had no choice but to have that sleep.

IRRITABLE BOWEL SYNDROME (IBS)

This unpleasant collection of bowel symptoms usually follows a cycle of 'flare-ups', often noted as worse under stress. The localised symptoms of constipation alternating with diarrhoea, coupled with abdominal pain, often with bloating, seem to generate other debilitating symptoms such as headache and tiredness. Many people seek help from nutritionists, and find that they have allergies and/or sensitivities to certain foods, so a certain amount of symptom control can be gained from avoidance of these. Learning AT most certainly helps the stress component, but your therapist will want to be certain that proper investigations have been undergone, in order to exclude any underlying pathology. Again, working on repressed anger may well be a significant factor in the healing process.

Case 1 — John
Aged 38, John led a busy life, working in the City, and bringing up three young children. His IBS flared up every two to three months, regardless of the care he took with his diet. He realised that it was a post-stress reaction, flaring up after a difficult period rather than during it. As he took on board the notion that it was letting go of stress which allowed the symptom out, he

decided to substitute Intentional Exercises for his symptoms. It worked — regular safe angry outbursts in private gave vent to pent-up feelings, while AT exercises gave his body and mind time for regular 'holidays' three tines a day. His symptoms improved markedly by the end of the course.

Case 2 — Theresa

A 28-year-old nurse, Theresa suffered 'bites' of IBS every six weeks or so. She recognised the contribution that childhood anger had made to her symptoms when, during her AT, she encountered upsetting memories from her past. The combination of relaxation (raising awareness) and using Intentional Off-loading Exercises helped her to regain control and reduce her symptoms.

OBESITY

When it comes to the need to lose weight, nothing can replace a good diet, re-education of eating habits, and physical exercise. However, AT can help the frame of mind in which these tasks are carried out. Sometimes insights are gained about why eating has been so out of kilter with good health. Low self-esteem and confidence are usually contributory factors, and if these are addressed through AT, the scene might be set to make positive physical change. Suppressed anger is often at the root of over-eating. Many of our clients have become aware that they are better able to be spontaneous in saying what they feel, and in allowing anger out rather than swallowing it (helped down by inappropriate eating).

PEPTIC ULCER

'What's eating you?' This question most eloquently describes the stomach ulcer. Anger and anxiety will most probably be the psychological link here. If we sit on our feelings, swallowing them down, our distress can increase acidity in the stomach, eventually causing ulceration. Recent research has identified the *helicobacter pylori* bacterium virus as the cause of some ulcers, which nowadays are treated with antibiotics. Maybe the person with recurring peptic ulcers needs to learn AT in order to break the cycle.

ENDOCRINE SYSTEM

DIABETES MELLITUS

Diabetes is a condition where the pancreas is unable to produce enough insulin for the body to deal with its sugar intake. If it is not treated, diabetes can be a serious life-threatening illness, especially when diagnosed in a young person. In this case it is usually described as 'insulin-dependent', and sufferers need to monitor themselves regularly for excess levels of sugar in their blood and urine, injecting themselves with insulin daily. When it is diagnosed in later life, it can usually be treated with oral medication and careful diet (non-insulin dependent).

Permanent adaptation is needed in lifestyle and diet, so it is inevitable that there is an emotional effect of developing diabetes. AT can help a person with diabetes to adjust to living with the condition, as well as helping the body to cope with treatment. Luthe's research showed positive results of improved response to insulin. In non-insulin dependent diabetes, AT can support the body's production of natural insulin.

It is vital for continued health that someone with diabetes takes responsibility for their own health, and collaborates with their physicians. AT encourages feelings of self-worth and confidence, which enables a person to get the best care for themselves. It gives tools to deal with emotional issues, and keeps stress levels under control.

An autogenic therapist will want to be confident that a diabetic person is carefully monitoring their blood-sugar levels during an AT course, as insulin requirements may change.

The complications associated with poorly managed diabetes play a significant part in the future of the person's health. Damage can be caused to many systems of the body, including: peripheral circulation, the kidneys and the eyes.

Case 1 — Lucy

Lucy, a single parent and a health worker, had been an insulin-dependent diabetic since childhood. Her stressful work and lifestyle contributed to difficulty in maintaining a stable blood sugar. She had recently experienced several severe hypoglycaemic attacks. Lucy was anxious about her long-term health. She hoped that AT would help her to gain control over her stress response. She felt frustrated by her lack of control over her body, and wanted to do something to help herself. Lucy monitored her own blood-sugar levels and informed her doctor of her attendance on the course.

From early on in the course, she experienced a number of discharges, including nausea and fatigue, which she related to her past physical and emotional experiences with diabetes. Lucy was, at first, resistant to the Intentional Off-loading Exercises — she had learnt how to 'cope' and not 'give in' to her emotions. She was surprised when she did engage with these exercises how much emotional material she was able to discharge, and the relief that this gave her. Her blood-sugar levels gradually stabilised, and her need for insulin decreased. Lucy also reported sleeping better and feeling less tense. At the follow-up session, she reported that her cholesterol levels had reduced, and she could think of no reason for this other than the effects of doing AT.

THYROID DISEASE

The potential for AT to help the body return to normal functioning can be supportive in both underactive and overactive thyroid problems, although any changes are likely to be slow. Several examples of research are in Luthe's books, showing the gradual reduction of protein–bound iodine (the old measurement of thyroid function) in thyrotoxicosis. AT can also help to improve troublesome symptoms, especially those exacerbated by stress.

GLANDULAR FEVER

Case 1 — Michael

Michael had been ill with glandular fever at the age of 32, and then returned to work, gradually building up his hours to full-time. He began to get recurrences of the illness, which is an accepted phenomenon of it. However, his symptoms had a pattern of their own: he would return from work on Fridays with a temperature of 103°, spend the weekend 'eating' paracetamol, then go back to work on Mondays. His wife had learned AT and insisted that he do so too. From the very first AT session, Michael's consumption of paracetamol ceased, and he was immediately able to enjoy weekends and family life.

Case 2 — Jeremy

Jeremy's glandular fever was supposedly a thing of the past. He had recovered, but, after a few months, he had to take at least a week off work — sometimes more — every two months, with recurrences of his symptoms. There were no recurrences during his AT course, and, after four months, his health remained excellent.

HEADACHES

GENERAL HEADACHES

We can suffer a headache for no apparent reason, but they are often referred to as 'tension headaches'.

Case 1 — Susan

A 50-year-old teacher, with two grown-up children, Susan had suffered headaches for many years. She thought nothing of taking Solpadeine on a daily basis. After some years, her doctor recommended that she learn AT. She reported in the fifth week of the nine-week course that she hadn't taken any Solpadeine at all since starting her Autogenic Training. 'I decided to have my headaches instead of fight them, and they disappeared.' Her medication (self-prescribed) dropped from eight tablets per day to none at all.

Case 2 — Brian

Brian was experiencing almost daily headaches while at work. He enjoyed his job but his work environment was very stressful — noisy, with constant interruptions. He was concerned about the amount of pain-relief he was using, and joined an AT group. After three weeks, his headaches became less frequent and less severe. As a bonus, his blood pressure, which had been slightly raised, returned to normal, and his sleep improved. He was able to concentrate more easily at work, and found himself enjoying life.

MIGRAINE HEADACHES

Chris Pinch worked on a project funded by a local health authority to test the efficacy of complementary therapy in general, and AT in particular, on migraine (See Chapter 12). The clients were selected from those who had not responded well to conventional treatment or who were on high doses of expensive medication. Overall, the results were excellent, showing reduction in frequency and severity of attacks. By the end of the trial, some people had gone for six months without an attack. Most had found benefit from feeling more in control. Many people found that they became more aware of what triggered their symptoms, or that they became more resistant or resilient to them.

Case 1 — Monica

Monica, at 55, had suffered very severe migraine for twenty-five years. She had 'tried' and studied several alternative approaches, all to some good effect, but unfortunately not permanent. She found herself feeling addicted to pain-killing medication for fear of a headache taking hold. Her life was always extremely busy, which was how she liked it — combining a rich artistic life with her carer's job. Over the years she had done a lot of therapeutic work on herself, and gained many insights, and still she had her migraines.

During the AT course, Monica's symptoms did not shift much, and, at the follow-up session, she reported that the previous day she had felt so low, and the pain had been so intense, that she had felt like crying. At the suggestion of her therapist (that this was a clear indication that she should indeed cry), she decided to use the Intentional Crying Exercise one weekend. The exercise developed into real crying, and she found that she 'went a bit deeper', recognising that she had neglected an important part of two grieving processes. After that, she found that her symptoms were much less intrusive, to the extent that for three weeks she was headache-free. Cautiously optimistic, she realised that she now has a new grief — that the answer (allowing herself to examine old grief and express it) was so simple that she could have saved herself a lot of agony.

Case 2 — Patricia

Patricia was in her fifties, and had become almost a total recluse because of her fear of a migraine attack. She had once been rendered helpless by migraine, while out on a trip, and she had felt humiliated by having to ask for help from strangers. Although her attacks were no more frequent than every six weeks, she would not commit herself to any social or community activity, staying at home most of the time 'in case' a migraine came on.

During the AT course, Patricia's fear of migraine receded — she was able to accept that others would not blame her for being ill and that she could cope with such eventualities. She used the Intentional Verbalisation of Anxiety Exercise to enhance the work of the Standard Exercises. She did not have a migraine at all while doing the course; she arranged social events without feeling the need to explain herself if she had to cancel; she had confidence that she would cope even if further attacks did occur.

Case 3 — Simon

Simon had suffered a severe head injury in a road-traffic accident two years before he came to learn AT, which had left him virtually incapacitated with almost daily migraines. He had lost his job as a result. He admitted to being very short-tempered at home, and was concerned about the effect of this on his family. He said that his quality of life was zero. He was desperate to improve things, yet conventional treatment had offered no solution.

Simon was well motivated and he practised diligently. After a few sessions, he reported feeling more relaxed generally, with less severe migraine attacks. Then he began to notice that some days were completely headache-free. By the end of the course, he was having only one or two episodes a week, which were much less intense. He was using markedly less medication, had taken up a favourite hobby again, was helping around the house, and had greatly improved relationships within the family.

Case 4 — Paula

A married woman of 48 who worked in the home, supporting her disabled husband, and as 'resident' baby-sitter for her seven grandchildren, Paula was recommended by her GP to learn AT. Her headaches 'attacked' twice a month or more, laying her low in bed for two or three days each time. Her GP often administered pethidine injections in the middle of the night. The court case regarding compensation for her husband's accident at work was still pending after nine years, causing untold distress. When questioned about her lifestyle of never-ending giving to others, her permanent smile spread: 'Oh, I love it. I love 'em. They're my life. I'm not complaining.' So, she was not complaining, but her head certainly was.

Paula loved the course. She developed a somewhat 'gung-ho' approach to the autogenic exercises, feeling that she was, at last, taking a positive step in gaining control of herself. In the second week, Paula reported that her headaches had 'got worse'. This turned out to be because she was overdoing her

AT practice. She listened more carefully to the instructions, practised as recommended, and stopped allowing her grand-children to enhance the feeling of heaviness by sitting on her.

Paula began to realise that her headaches were a form of stress-release, that they provided her with an opportunity to take a break from the stress around her. She felt encouraged by her new perception, and felt that it was safe to encourage that release using AT.

She denied her anger: 'I haven't time to be angry.' The next week, she *was* angry, about how her family treated her home, and she realised that some of this had come about because she had allowed it to. 'I'm a big softy and I love them, but now I feel so angry.' The following week, she reported that she had used the Intentional Verbalisation Anger exercise in private. Then she called a family meeting, talked to all her children, collected in her house keys, told them to phone before arriving, and negotiated baby-sitting to Fridays only, for the daughter who was most in need of her support.

'They were all fine about it.' Paula was surprised. All those years she had never thought about what her life was doing to her — and when she finally did, and took action, nobody minded. Perhaps the biggest surprise was that she had never thought of standing up for herself. She had gone on in the same old patterns, regardless of the effect on her health.

So what happened to her headaches? They had not disappeared. If anything, they were slightly more frequent, but much less severe. Pethidine was never mentioned. She was encouraged by the changing pattern of her symptoms, and was even glad that they hadn't disappeared altogether. They were now a measure of what was going on and how she was coping.

By the end of the nine weeks, Paula was planning a holiday — the first in years. She had always been too frightened that a headache would 'attack' during it. 'What about your headaches while you're away?' Her answer was almost serene, no longer defensive. 'Oh, I'll take them with me — packed in the suitcase.'

Immune System Disorders

Acquired Immune Deficiency Syndrome (AIDS)

The disease involves the infiltration of the immune system by the Human Immunodeficiency Virus (HIV), which lives and reproduces in the system. In a HIV-positive person, the virus is dormant and inactive. If the person develops AIDS itself, the immune response weakens, and is unable to cope with infections, eventually leading to death through several 'AIDS-related' diseases. In the mid–1980s, one of our colleagues, Dr Kai Kermani, used AT in this area with some very positive outcomes.

Dr Kermani found that the quality of life improved dramatically in those with HIV or AIDS, when they learned AT. It helped the devastating perception that their lives and health were spiralling out of control. Treatment was combined with other complementary approaches: diet, vitamin and mineral supplements, and specific forms of meditation. This is a good example of how AT is used in conjunction with other treatments, to improve both health and life expectancy.

Obviously we make no claims to cure, but there is no doubt that AT will play its part in the healing process. Also, for those whose condition will be terminal, the autogenic principles of trusting the body's processes, along with using the Intentional Exercises, allows a peaceful transition in the journey of dying.

Inefficient Immune System

Case 1 — Leslie

A married man of 32, with a 3-year-old daughter, Leslie had suffered recurring throat infections and chest colds, requiring one or two weeks off sick in every four to six weeks. He joined an AT course in his workplace, and missed the second session because of another infection, but he found that he recovered more quickly than usual. He attended all remaining sessions, practising diligently, and then continued in excellent health. In this case alone, Autogenic Therapy created a large financial saving for his employers, in terms of lost time through sickness.

Case 2 — June

A 47-year-old mother of two, June was also the Head Teacher of a large comprehensive school. She learned AT to help deal with the stressful demands of her job, and hoped for better general health as a result. She did her course during the autumn term, and was delighted to report that she escaped the coughs and colds which all her staff were suffering around her. For the first time in her career, she reached Christmas without any illness or time off work, relishing her increased energy.

Case 3 — Rupert

A busy GP of 38, Rupert learned AT as much out of curiosity as anything else. However, a few years later, he reported that he was now able to organise his holidays so that he could travel on the day after he left work. Previously, he had always left two or three days to 'unwind' and allow any stress-related colds, coughs or stomach upsets to emerge and clear before he travelled. He changed this habit when he realised that he was sitting at home 'on holiday' for no reason other than fear of non-existent symptoms!

LIFE–THREATENING ILLNESS

The distress, anxiety and feelings of helplessness surrounding terminal illness are an inevitable part of it, and this is one area where AT can help enormously. We would make no claim that AT could effect a cure, but it is, however, invaluable in enhancing the effects of conventional treatment (drug therapy, radiotherapy and recovery from surgery). If the situation is clearly a terminal one, AT can help the person to ease their way forward towards a gentle release into death. AT would also be of great help for the carers of terminally ill people — to cope with their distress, fatigue and emotions during these times.

CANCER
AT has been used for many years in specialist centres such as the
Bristol Cancer Help Centre and the Wirral Holistic Care Centre.
It contributes to the development of a positive attitude of mind,
and to a more efficient immune-system functioning.

Changing Attitudes
Much research has been done which claims to have identified the
'cancer personality'. The person who lives a striving and non-stop
life, always 'doing' for others, and not standing up for themselves,
with no room for contemplation, recharging batteries, or expression of emotions, may have an increased risk of cancer developing.
The person who recognises their true worth, and their own
limitations, and is not afraid of their feelings will have a natural
defence against cancer.

When serious illness has taken hold, AT often helps to create a
new perspective and balance. In the case of completed treatment,
the mind and body will be better able to maintain this, with the
'clean slate' of good health. Usually, as part of their autogenic
process, the person needs to acknowledge and work through the
negative feelings (often fear and/or anger) associated with their
illness and treatment.

Case 1 — Malcolm
Malcolm was 54 when his cancer (of the bowel) was diagnosed. He had just left his job with much relief as, for the sake
of his family, he had spent his whole working life in an unrewarding career which did not interest him. He looked
forward to satisfying his creative talents and starting a new
career in writing. However, he had to have major surgery followed by radiotherapy, which was, of course, devastating. He
decided to learn AT after his recovery.

The early stages of Malcolm's autogenic process were
extremely difficult for him — he described quite disturbing
intruding thoughts. These were linked with anxiety about his

---

health. He became obsessed that his thoughts would cause his cancer to recur. He was desperate to find distraction from them, but in the autogenic state he could not escape them. 'My thoughts are crying out to me.' These words (his) graphically describe what was happening. The autogenic process was bringing his anxiety to the fore, whether he liked it or not. The course was in its earliest stages, and his therapist wished to let the process unfold without plunging too soon into using Intentional Off-loading Exercises. However, she encouraged him to cut back his AT to short-stitch exercises, and to use his writing skills to allow the feelings out on paper, which might lead on to crying and a considerable degree of feeling upset. Then he should symbolically tear it up. She explained how the imbalance of logic versus feeling needed redressing, and the autogenic exercises were making that happen. The logical left-brain hemisphere knew that his treatment had been successful — but the right-brain hemisphere had catching-up to do — it was still locked in unexpressed fear.

Malcolm persevered with his AT, and eventually was able to tolerate other thoughts during it, while working on them outside the exercises. Gradually he realised that he had never grieved for the loss of his good health, or expressed his feelings about the possibility of death. In the following weeks, he addressed all this in his Off-loading Exercises, and ended the course feeling very much more positive. He was aware that his good health was not assured, but he was not so afraid of his feelings, and was certain that he would be able to cope with whatever the future held.

Case 2 — Maggie

Maggie completed her AT course at the second attempt — early in the first course, a diagnosis of breast cancer was confirmed and she had immediate surgery. When she returned two years later, she told her therapist the story of her journey. During her chemotherapy treatment, she had been very ill, but nevertheless had decided to organise a Christmas celebration with her whole family, knowing that it might be her last one. Her children, all aware of her condition, gathered from different parts of the globe and country, and they had a moving and open time together. It was another year before Maggie, now given the 'all-clear', resumed and completed her AT.

Maggie worked well with all aspects of the course, from which she drew a great deal of emotional strength. She was grateful to AT for enhancing her new insights about herself and her health. She now had no fear about dying; she had communicated a great deal to her family; she was at peace with herself and her life.

Musculo-Skeletal Tension

If the muscles are holding a great deal of tension, it is hard to shift pain. The cause of the pain also needs to be established — AT can't fix everything! We both recommend osteopathy or certain forms of chiropractic in order to help an acute problem. When chronic pain recurs, despite successful treatment, there may be an element of 'holding on' to it. Learning to let go in terms of muscle tension can result in pain-free life.

We have found that our clients often report that their masseur, osteopath or chiropractor notices that it is easier to give them a treatment now that they are able to relax. In other words, this is a clear instance of how AT will enhance treatment from other therapies. The mind and body are more receptive to it, so it will be more effective. Many of our clients report that they need to go for other treatment less frequently than they used to.

Back Pain; Frozen Shoulder; Neck Pain

These problems are some of the commonest causes of absenteeism from work. Clearly, attention needs to be paid to posture and use of equipment, but a chronic condition of back pain can very often be improved with AT. The psychosomatic element of these pains cannot be ignored. As stress builds, muscular tension rises, and because we are not in the habit of paying attention to our bodies, we notice this only when pain results. Once they have learned to focus on their bodies, the majority of our clients become aware of neck and shoulder tension being present. This is easily corrected with the simplest of AT exercises.

MYALGIC ENCEPHALOMYELITIS; FATIGUE SYNDROMES

These illnesses 'of our times' have caused much debate in medical and psychological circles. Is 'ME' ('yuppie flu' used to be its disparaging name) a pathological disease (illness) or is it 'all in the mind'? A UK government report published in January 2002 states that it is a genuine illness. Some complementary practitioners believe that the immune systems of sufferers have been damaged by certain types of vaccinations. The authors find that those who come to learn AT are usually harbouring a considerable amount of repressed anger, linking with previous life events. Who is to say that the conversion of that anger into depression isn't the trigger which causes the mind–body response to develop ME? This would tie in with other distressing symptoms which go with the physical pain and fatigue.

ME and chronic-fatigue sufferers will always tell you about their frustrations when doctors tell them that their problems are caused by depression. Their reply is: *'I wasn't depressed before — wouldn't you be depressed if you had this illness?'*.

AT usually helps a great deal. It is not always about 'being cured' (although if the person has reached the point where recovery is near, AT is likely to speed this up) but we would estimate that 90 per cent of sufferers appreciate the help it has given in coping with the illness, most especially in being able to rest more effectively and manage their energy levels better.

Case 1 — Elizabeth
Elizabeth had suffered from ME for eight years. An intelligent woman, she had had to give up her teaching career because, at times, she was wheel-chair-bound, and she wanted to devote

---

whatever energy she had to her young family. During her AT course, she discovered that she had issues regarding her relationship with her mother, which had coloured most of her life choices. Through using Intentional Exercises, she resolved a lot of this, improved her current relationships, and was delighted to report after six months that her ME symptoms had all but disappeared. In this case it was likely that her spontaneous recovery had already been well underway, and AT had helped to speed it up.

Case 2 — Marion

Marion, 25, had been married for only a year when her ME began. This was in the days where she could not find a doctor who would believe her, which of course put a great strain on her new marriage. Eventually she found AT through a homoeopathic doctor, and underwent a group course. At the end of the nine weeks, and the follow-up (a total period of four months), she said that she was disappointed not to have made more inroads into her physical symptoms. However, she was delighted that she had gained a lot of insight into the emotional components of her illness — and she had learned a 'box of tricks' to help her to cope.

Case 3 — Harry

A young and formerly very fit young man of 28, Harry was extremely angry. His illness had meant that he had had to give up all his sporting activities (some of which were at national competition level), and he was feeling desperate about his failing energy and health. He found AT hard to do — his whole demeanour was used to focusing on action and achievement. He rejected the use of the Intentional Exercises (even though the anger exercise is enormously helpful in these circumstances), and in the end he rejected AT. Perhaps the timing was wrong for him.

NEUROLOGICAL DISORDERS

EPILEPSY

Improvement in the number of fits will vary according to the frequency and severity of their occurrence. If fits are rare, it may take several years to find out whether there has been any improvement. Your therapist will always liaise with your medical consultant, and it is vital that you continue your medication — discuss stopping it only with careful monitoring. Again, AT is extremely useful for reducing anxiety about symptoms, and the general distress about being epileptic.

Case 1 — Sue

Aged 42, Sue worked as an administrator for a boss who neither treated her well, nor, in her opinion, did his job at all adequately, giving rise to much frustration in her life. In addition, when she first enquired about AT, Sue had recently suffered a fit which had not been completely investigated. It was suggested that she might have epilepsy, but eventually she was diagnosed with Arterial-Venous Malformation in her right frontal lobe. Understandably she was extremely anxious about the situation, and also depressed, with thoughts about life not being worth living, and yet she feared that she might die.

Treatment was offered via a special angiogram, and in the event she underwent this after seven weeks of AT — and she was back at work in a week. Post-operatively Sue felt very unsettled, with poor sleep and a lot of unpleasant dreams. She felt unable to 'get into' her AT, and did not think of using Intentional Off-loading Exercises. In time, she recovered, and overall she knew that AT had helped her cope with this situation. Her scores about her life rose dramatically from her assessment, and she found new energy and determination to seek a new job. Being unsure of a new direction she used the personal formula: 'Possibilities are my purpose' because she felt that a lack of purpose had always held her back.

MULTIPLE SCLEROSIS

The threat of progressive disability is what usually brings MS sufferers to learn AT. A sense of urgency not to 'be beaten' by the illness is coupled with a need to try to prevent the situation from getting worse. No one can predict whether AT might be instrumental in this prevention since it is well known that the degree of degeneration varies enormously. Some people can descend to being bedridden, while others may spend the rest of their lives 'in remission'. All we can say is that AT has the potential to help the distressing anxieties, frustrations and grief surrounding the diagnosis. Our clients with MS who have learned AT invariably report feeling better able to cope with the circumstances of their illness and the limitations of their lives.

NEURALGIA

Trigeminal neuralgia affects the facial nerves and causes severe sharp pains in the side of the face and head. The person usually recognises their own triggers for it. AT often helps to reduce the frequency and severity — probably by reducing the attendant fear of the symptom. A positive attitude of acceptance can contribute to symptom reduction.

PARKINSON'S DISEASE

As with all diseases of a progressive nature, the emotional aspects of the illness can feel as 'desperate' as the physical ones of losing control because of the characteristic tremors and 'freezing' spasms of the limbs. AT has long been recognised as being of particular help in reducing stress, which in turn helps the tension associated with tremor and spasm. Recent research by Professor Leader (who works with his nutritionist wife and with our colleague, Vera Diamond), suggests that the relaxation of AT is instrumental in increasing levels of dopamine in the brain, thereby actively contributing to the treatment of the disease. However, great motivation is needed by the client, with a willingness to work with all aspects of the method, especially the Intentional Exercises regarding anger (frustration) and crying (grief).

Case 1 — Barbara

Aged 54, Barbara had been diagnosed with Parkinson's eleven years previously. In the last two years, her symptoms had worsened to the extent that she was virtually confined to a wheelchair when she left the house. The strain was telling on her husband, who, with the best will in the world, wanted to support her, but was increasingly suffering from exhaustion. In addition to her difficulties in walking, Barbara also suffered severe neck tension, especially if she went to the theatre — she realised this was partly a result of the self-consciousness she felt in a public place.

Both Barbara and her husband learned AT, but neither really engaged with the very real necessity to deal with their feelings. Barbara's husband remained in his role of 'cheering her up', while Barbara would continue to give vent to her anger with him present, rather than safely when he was out playing golf. At the end of the course, both acknowledged that AT had helped them, that they probably hadn't really given it a 'proper chance', and that Barbara was sleeping a great deal better.

PHANTOM-LIMB PAIN

In our experience, AT is not used specifically for this — amputation may have been part of the client's history, but they are learning AT for something else.

Case 1 — Neil

An army sergeant, Neil had read about AT as a useful means to improve sports, so JB was surprised to meet a man who had had a below-knee amputation (war wounds nine years previously). He succeeded in winning all kinds of pistol-shooting competitions in the end, but at the start was uncertain why JB was concerned about his possible adverse reactions to the heaviness exercise. In the event, he surprised himself by how in touch with his missing leg he still was. After Neil's questioning of the wording of the exercise ('How can I say "My right leg is heavy" when half of it isn't there?'), JB had suggested that he find his own way. However, when he used the phrase, he found that his right leg was just as 'present' as the left. There was no pain, but the comforting presence helped his general healing.

STAMMERING

It is usually the accompanying embarrassment of stammering which can contribute to the severity of the symptom. So, if AT can reduce the level of attendant anxiety, a degree of success is already present. As usual, we would make no promises as to outcome, because many different causative factors will have played their part. It is commonly understood that where left-handed tendencies have been squashed in childhood, a stammer is likely to result. AT needs to be taught with no emphasis at all given to the problem. A stammering child may or may not respond well to AT alone. Treatment needs to be given in conjunction with other agencies, such as speech therapy, or play therapy.

STROKES

Provided that the stroke is not too severe, AT will help the rehabilitation progress after it. A determined person will use all the tools available in the AT course to help themselves. As ever, Intentional Exercises are invaluable in helping with the expression of feelings. If the speech centre is affected, it doesn't matter — making any sound will help to release the feelings. As strength is recovered, hitting pillows can be immensely rewarding in releasing frustration.

PREGNANCY AND CHILDBIRTH

Over the years, much research has been done showing AT to be an extremely valuable asset in pregnancy and labour. Certainly it is Jane Bird's great regret that she had not discovered AT before the births of her three children. Any relaxation is wonderful in pregnancy, of course. Using AT carries that extra special message of knowing that you are giving your baby the best and calmest experience in the womb. It is possible to use all the Standard Exercises, although attention is paid to the reaction to the cardiac-regulation exercise

— sometimes palpitations can be exacerbated by it. Also, we tend to leave the abdominal warmth exercise out — the mother's body will do its own adapting, and therapists acknowledge that if certain problems occur in pregnancy, especially any that might cause haemorrhage, the abdominal warmth exercise might not help it.

However, AT helps to build up confidence and psychological strength before facing labour and birth; it helps by providing a tool-kit of 'tricks' to use between contractions; it helps to alleviate pain; it helps to maintain an attitude of 'getting on with it' with a feeling of control; and it helps recovery after delivery. Post-delivery sleep preceded by an AT exercise will be more profound than 'ordinary' sleep. And think of all those night-time feeds: AT will help you to get back to sleep afterwards. Or you might have a restless colicky baby — the neck and shoulders formula is a godsend, helping your patience and stamina. As you use AT, even if just simple, partial exercises, you will communicate the positive attitude to the baby. What a start to their life!

Case 1 — Annette

Annette, aged 40, a complementary therapist, was pregnant with her first child from her second marriage. From her first marriage, she already had a 13-year-old son, whom she had brought up on her own. Annette was concerned not only about undergoing labour at her age, but also about the effect the new baby might have on her son and the whole family dynamic. She wanted to give her new baby 'the best start' and reduce her tendency to be snappy and irritable. She started the course at thirty-two weeks pregnant, and completed only heaviness, warmth and breathing. She delivered two weeks early, without the Caesarean section she had been warned might be necessary. She managed everything more calmly than she had thought she would, and was very impressed that her new son was calm, not at all restless and 'niggly', despite the relative trauma of needing a suction 'cap' to aid his delivery.

Case 2 — Nikki Bradford, Health Writer
(Nikki is a great supporter of AT and gave us permission to use her name and story.)

After the birth of her first baby, Nikki didn't have an unbroken night's sleep for two years, waking for the baby two or three times a night. 'I continued my journalism career working from home, trying to write, and I began to fall apart. I went on a sleep training course for the baby, which was wonderfully successful. But then I discovered I still couldn't sleep — I would lie awake waiting for the baby to wake!' Once, at 3.45 a.m. Nikki found herself about to bang her head against the wall, and she decided to do something about it. She phoned around and found AT, which 'seemed both sensible and practical'. She slept after the very first session, which she certainly didn't expect.

Nikki became pregnant with her second child one year later. She wasn't looking forward to it as her first labour had been very long. She used personal and motivational formulae in her AT: 'Smoothly, labour quick and efficient'; 'My body remembers what to do;' 'It will be all right', etc. When her time came, her labour stopped after she was admitted to hospital. She heard a lot of crying and pain from other patients and, using AT, told herself, 'It will not be like this'.

She found that by using AT, she needed no painkillers; the lights were low, and her husband supported her by repeating the autogenic and personal phrases for her. Suddenly she thought, 'Yes — I remember this!' and felt no fear as the medical staff broke her waters. The baby was born five minutes later!

Nikki knows that AT helped to keep her centred, yet calm. She was calm while pregnant, and after the birth, and able to make the most of her rest periods. Best of all, she slept. She is well aware, from her own experience, of how AT is very likely to prevent post-natal depression.

Applications of Autogenic Therapy

INFERTILITY

It is a well-known fact that stress and anxiety are the cause of many delayed successes in conception. Our lifestyles demand too much of us. And we expect to be able to time what should be a completely natural event. So, the pressure is huge for the poor old sperm to make its mark on a particular day, so that the baby's birth coincides with the company's end of financial year (for example)! There is no doubt that AT can help a woman to become pregnant when there is no gynaecological reason why she shouldn't. AT may help some minor imbalances of her hormones, as well as bringing about a more relaxed attitude. For that matter, AT can help the man too — in both cases probably by bringing about a state of mind that is more laid back and accepting that what will be will be. We both have stories of women who, at the initial assessment, expressed disappointment at the time it was taking to get pregnant — and by the follow-up session were booking into the ante-natal clinic!

Case 1 — Jenny

Aged 27, and married for about four years, Jenny was keen to start a family, but was disappointed and worried that she had problems. Having stopped using contraception a year previously, she was not pregnant. She was going through monthly cycles of disappointment, which were compounding into quite severe anxiety about her perceived failing reproductive system. Her doctor had suggested that she learn to relax, which was why she had joined the course. During the fourth session she told her therapist that she was 90 per cent sure that she was pregnant. The implication was that she had conceived before she even started AT — after the initial assessment. Clearly, the first step to doing something positive had broken the cycle of worry.

> Case 2 — Sally
>
> Sally was 33, and her anxiety about getting pregnant was paramount. She had been married for eight years, and had a high-powered job, which she did not want to give up, but she did want to have a baby. Her ambivalence about her work contributed to her dilemma. Also, she had had two terminations of pregnancy in her late teens, and was seriously concerned that she had ruined her chances of pregnancy. She had discussed none of this with her husband — feeling too ashamed at her past behaviour. Her AT process included a lot of self-examination, including the realisation that she needed to grieve for her two lost babies. She also managed to talk to her husband, allowing her fears and guilt to surface. Three months later, she was pregnant, glowing and happy. She reported that she probably wouldn't return to her current job, but would find something more family-friendly when she was ready.

POST-NATAL DEPRESSION

This most distressing occurrence comes at a particularly important time in both the new mother's and the new baby's life. Just when the bonding is getting established, the mother finds that she can't cope, feels anxious, tearful and exhausted all the time, and, in some cases, might be in danger of harming herself or her baby. No one knows the absolute reason for PND, but we should not ignore all the contributory factors surrounding childbirth.

The mother's hormones will have been truly disturbed for the best part of a year. This will affect the mind (attitudes, fears, behaviour, etc.) of course. But we, the authors, wonder if other factors are not given the prominence they should receive. Particularly when you have a first baby, the shock to the system is huge — you can never prepare for it. That shock is both physical (the body has undergone the most enormous event of its life) and emotional (the life-change which begins from the very first moment of conception will be relentless for the next 20+ years). These aspects need to be acknowledged and addressed.

First, a process of grief needs to be undergone. Even though the pregnancy and delivery have been untoward, and all is well, this huge life-change must be dealt with on an emotional level. You, the mother, need to have that traditional 'fifth-day baby blues' loud and clear. The unexplained tears need to pour, and you should be allowed to be able *not* to cope for a few hours. Through doing this, the realisation will dawn that: '*This is my life from now on*'; '*I have lost my old life*'. You will ask yourself, '*How am I going to cope?*' There will be elements of sadness for the loss, followed by anger and frustration at this little scrap of humanity being utterly dependent, and probably ruling your life. You may feel angry with yourself: '*What have I done?*'

The important thing is to be honest about your feelings. Of course, you are delighted with your baby — you have been excitedly preparing for months. This is all that you have been waiting for. So all these negative feelings are most unwelcome. If you deny them, pasting a smile on to hide your feelings, and you never let your truthful tears and angst out, you are more likely to develop PND later. Of course, a supportive partner, with whom you can share your feelings, will also play a major part in preventing PND.

Perhaps in the old days of extended families, there was enough support for this to happen. Nowadays, mothers may be left to their own devices more than previously. Warning them in advance that they will need to do this might help, but all mothers we have spoken to have said things like: '*Why didn't someone tell me what it would be like?*' Someone probably did, but prospective mothers don't listen — nature's way of protecting the human race!

Using AT will help you to allow this natural process of emotional release after childbirth to happen quite spontaneously. In addition, you will have the confidence and trust in your own processes to go along with it, without suppressing the feelings.

Case 1 — Caroline

Aged 34, Caroline was the mother of a 3-year-old boy, and was now twelve weeks pregnant with her second child. She had suffered post-natal depression for a year after the first baby, feeling completely unsupported by her husband and family. In fact, feelings of this nature are quite normal, but when she became tearful and unable to cope, everyone around her told her that she 'shouldn't feel like that' — she was 'so lucky to have a healthy baby'. So she became anxious that she wasn't normal, which caused feelings of inadequacy and worthlessness. Medication helped, as did the growing up of her son. She was afraid of this happening again and was determined to prevent it.

During the AT pre-course assessment, various family issues came to light, and she realised that she had been brought up never to complain — speaking about feelings (let alone expressing them) was a 'no-no' in her parents' house. As the process unfolded, Caroline understood that, after her first child had been born, she had felt frightened and alone, but she had told no one. She also understood that if she had opened up, at least to her husband early on, things might have turned out differently. But the biggest revelation was the surprise that she should have grieved for her previous life, after the baby was born. So she did, during her AT course. The result was a more aware pregnancy and labour, and a willingness to acknowledge her truthful feelings with her husband later. No more PND!

Psychological Problems

Anxiety/Panic Attacks

Anxiety, as we have seen earlier, is an important warning signal for us. When we are in danger, the adrenaline response kicks in and we notice a dry mouth, cold and sweaty hands and feet, a racing heart, fast 'panting' breathing. All of these physiological changes are a positive help to us, if we need to be alert to danger, and prepared to run or fight.

However, this is a primeval physiological response which, in our modern lives, does not carry the same relevance as it did when we were fending for ourselves in the jungle. These days, we can get caught up in habitual anxiety — a free-floating, non-specific anxiety without recognisable cause. If this develops into a full-blown panic attack, it can be very frightening — indeed, many people report that they feel as though they are going to die.

This can be very debilitating, as the constant fear restricts our lifestyles and decreases our quality of life. Activities or situations are avoided, narrowing down a person's life to uncomfortable limits. Anxiety feelings may have been precipitated by a traumatic event. Perhaps we learn anxious attitudes from our parents. Sometimes the label 'anxious personality' is applied, giving rise to the question of whether it is inherited (genetic), or acquired (environmental influences). People often say: 'If I don't have something to worry about, I worry until I've found something.' In Italy, research by Professor Farné found that, after learning AT, people with long-standing anxiety showed a reversal of these tendencies (see Chapter 12) .

AT is generally wonderful for anxiety — whatever form it takes. During the Standard Exercises, the sympathetic branch of the autonomic nervous system is quietened down, and the parasympathetic (to do with rest, recuperation and recovery) is activated. As you learn to do this at will, so you start to break the vicious circle which is the habit of anxiety. Once the off-loading and readjustment process has settled down, it should be clinically impossible to feel panic while in an autogenic state.

We have found that anxiety is often the 'face' of other repressed feelings. If someone has learned that anger is a 'bad thing', they have probably become afraid of it, giving rise to the vicious circles of anxiety. Those who have suffered a bereavement, and not been able to work adequately through their grief, are often left with feelings of anxiety. Once they get in touch with the grief feelings, and express them with the Intentional Off-loading Exercises, the anxiety subsides.

No claims or promises are ever made as to outcomes in AT. Both authors know of clients for whom their anxiety would not shift. But here we would suggest that it was playing its part in protecting the person — the feeling was alerting the client to issues which needed addressing, and sometimes, with the best will in the world, we as therapists cannot bring that about. The time is not always right. We have both known people to reach the end of the course without any alleviation of their anxiety symptoms, and yet they may phone a few months or years later to revisit their AT — perhaps stronger and better able to cope with the issues.

Case 1 — Barbara
In her late twenties, Barbara had a job as a speech therapist, which was very demanding yet rewarding. Her anxiety levels were very high, which disturbed much of her daily life. She knew that there were issues around from her childhood ('my parents were never available — I brought myself up') which had never been resolved, despite many attempts to do so. Barbara realised that her anxiety was a mask for her anger about the past, and she also acknowledged the grief for the loss of the loving family she had never had. A driven perfectionist, she realised that she would never get the approval of her parents, and tested this out by refusing to do any AT exercises one week. The therapist observed her process, making very little comment, and, by the end of the course, Barbara's anxiety had significantly reduced. She learned to respond to it in terms of what other feelings needed to be addressed.

Case 2 — Andrew
A 43-year-old financial director, Andrew had suffered symptoms of anxiety for twenty years, for which he used beta-blocker medication. By the end of his AT course, he had not taken any medication for five weeks, and his anxiety had all but disappeared. Even when he was aware of it on occasion, he could accept it, express his feelings about it, and it would

disappear. He had discovered that his anxiety was, in fact, triggered by feelings of anger or sadness, which he had previously tried to suppress. But that suppression meant that anxiety emerged instead.

Case 3 — Rosemary

This 23-year-old woman had suffered emotional trauma in a violent relationship and, as a reaction, had indulged in abusing non-prescribed drugs over a period of two years. ('You name it, I used it: Pot, Amphetamines, Cocaine, Ecstasy. It was fine — it was fun — I could conquer the world.') Then she had a very unpleasant experience with Ecstasy, from which she took a whole day to recover, and she vowed that she would never touch any such stuff ever again. She switched into severe anxiety, and found herself having great difficulties in eating or drinking normal food. Her breathing was also a cause for concern — she kept thinking that she couldn't breathe properly, and that she had to 'make myself breathe'. She sought help from her GP and, a few months later, started AT. There were a number of difficulties early on, when she experienced unpleasant reactions in the autogenic state, especially when she did exercises in bed at night, and the process needed to be slowed down. By the end of the course, she had released herself from the anxiety; she could manage AT exercises for sleep, which itself had improved; and her breathing had settled down to its natural rhythms again. Other issues in her past still needed addressing — or perhaps AT had led her to a place where she could simply let go and move on in her life.

Case 4 — Alison

Aged 47, Alison was in an impossible situation as regards her husband, from whom she was separated. They were still living in the same house, but he would never tell her his movements, so he could be away with his new partner but she wouldn't know until he came back. Neither would he proceed with the divorce and settlement so that they could sell the house. Still reliant on him for her income, she felt disinclined to provoke him by changing the locks. But she felt that she couldn't lead a normal life — for example, she couldn't have friends around in case he walked in and caused her to 'get in a state'. Very quickly, Alison was able to use AT to her advantage. It became her refuge, her private place of rest and recovery. As the weeks went by, she began to make remarks such as, 'I coped really well at my solicitor's this week.' And gleefully, 'My husband is amazed by the way I am staying calm in all this.' By the end of the course, her anxiety had disappeared, she was using Intentional Exercises (but not many) and the Standard Exercises, and she was relishing her new skills to take with her into her new life.

BEREAVEMENT AND UNRESOLVED GRIEF

As described in Chapter 5, the process of grief is often suppressed, giving rise to all kinds of difficulty. Grief is around many times in our lives — whether it be through bereavement when someone close to us dies, or loss of a job or of our good health. The process of grieving is often delayed, through fear of our own emotions, or (mistakenly) to protect others from theirs. We are adept at avoiding the grieving process by diverting ourselves with work or other activity. This may give rise to psychosomatic symptoms which can appear or persist many years after the initial loss, and which may have brought the person to learn AT. These symptoms can include: depression, headaches or migraine, unexplained aches and pains, anxiety, blocked sinuses and catarrh, runny nose (often known as allergic rhinitis), twitching eye muscles and facial tics, frequent tears, general fatigue.

Case 1 — Judy
Judy, a woman in her forties, whose mother had died six months previously, had been suffering from neuralgia (severe facial pain). Treatment was ineffective and the symptoms

returned. Judy had been close to her mother, and after her death had busied herself organising the funeral and sorting out her mother's affairs. Then she had buried herself in her own work. She acknowledged that she had never cried for her mother, and although she recognised the need, she was unable to let it happen. After several weeks of practising the Standard Exercises, episodes of crying began to occur spontaneously, and the Intentional Crying Exercise was introduced. At first, Judy did not find this easy, but she persisted, and her pain receded, then disappeared.

Case 2 — Pat

Pat was someone who had been practising AT for some time when her mother died. She knew that she should grieve, but she hadn't found it convenient to do so. She developed a pain in her shoulder blades, which she eventually suspected might be a crying-need symptom. She decided to use the Crying Exercise, and the pain disappeared.

Case 3 — Carol

Carol's mother had died three years before Carol came to learn AT. Her two children had been very small at the time, and Carol was now experiencing 'increasing problems with stress'. Thoughts of her mother arose in the early weeks of the course, and in the fourth week she complained of symptoms of hay fever (in January). She was advised to use the Intentional Crying Exercise, and her symptoms were relieved, only to reappear a few days later. With further use of the ICE, the symptoms completely disappeared, as eventually did her other 'stress'-related problems.

EATING DISORDERS (*ANOREXIA NERVOSA AND BULIMIA*)
We have often worked with clients with a past history of anorexia or bulimia — with interesting results.

Case 1 — Georgina

A 36-year-old financial adviser, Georgina was originally from continental Europe, and was looking forward to getting married to her English fiancé. She had suffered severe anorexia as a teenager, and was left with anxiety symptoms which she wanted to alleviate. After many months of psychotherapy, she now recognised that her symptoms were largely a reaction to her strict upbringing and her poor relationship with her mother, whom she described as domineering. After three weeks of AT, she described her disappointment that, despite great effort, she could feel herself slipping back into old eating patterns again. She had seen a nutritionist and was taking supplements, but she was worried that now she was vomiting the supplements up after breakfast. In a state of high anxiety, she discussed this with her therapist and the nutritionist involved.

It was clear that this was part of her autogenic process, especially as she described other 'good' things about AT. Despite her anxiety, she was sleeping better than she ever had. She was dreaming — much of it about her early life, re-encountering childhood scenarios involving her relationship with her mother. One day she became really angry, and used the Intentional Verbalisation of Aggression Exercise to off-load old feelings about her mother, recognising as she did so that she had had to leave her homeland as the only way to put distance between her mother and herself. Further discussion brought the realisation that she was grieving too — for the loss of the 'wished-for' mother she never had, and for the loss of her homeland.

Her nutritionist was impressed by the work Georgina was doing, and agreed that AT had temporarily 'tipped' her back into old habits. After all, the anorexia was the only method she knew to take control at the time, and it was always possible that this habit would return as an automatic kick-back at first. Time was needed for the re-balancing process to take effect, for her childhood feelings to be expressed, and then for her to be reassured by the certain knowledge that all was well — that she was now adult and removed from those difficulties. The best thing to do was to allow the process to continue, trusting that when it was worked through, her eating would return to the normal patterns which she had reached before. They did — within one week. By the end of the course, Georgina was very pleased that she had discovered a new honesty in herself, which had increased her self-confidence and improved her relationship with her fiancé.

This story is a powerful illustration of how AT can heal real distress. However, we are careful to point out that Georgina had already done a lot of preliminary work on the psychological aspects of her problems — her autogenic therapist had ascertained that anorexic symptoms had not been 'live' for fifteen years before starting AT.

PENT-UP AGGRESSION

There are constant aggravations in modern living. Our society is riddled with rage: road rage, air rage, supermarket rage. We are told that even queuing for the photocopier at work causes rage. Many of us bottle up our frustrations in our efforts to bring them under control. We are left with many symptoms and behavioural attitudes which we may confuse with our personality (*'It's just me'*), and we start to hate ourselves. Aggressive thoughts and actions, irritability and temper tantrums lead to exhaustion, restlessness, bad dreams, chest and abdominal pain, haemorrhoids, headaches, etc.

AT helps to address the issues and the feelings. Rather than hate themselves, the person is able to reduce their symptoms and release their anger through using AT exercises and the Intentional Verbalisation of Aggression Exercise. Often, issues of guilt are resolved, and the person emerges with new skills for dealing with their feelings, and with the possibility that anger is no longer needed. Perhaps it was a defence — a way of avoiding having to deal with life issues, or a significant relationship.

Case 1 — Frank
Frank came for AT because he was tired all the time, and had a lot of tension. When anger was discussed, he really didn't want to have anything to do with the Intentional Off-loading Exercises. As he spoke, saying that he had no problems with anger, he was hitting his fist into his other palm. After the end of the course, he rang his therapist to say that he was addicted to his relaxation exercises. If he didn't do his AT, he was like a bear with a sore head, snapping at everyone around him. After a further consultation and discussion around this, he began practising the Intentional Verbalisation of Anger Exercise. His general demeanour improved so much that he could even manage without doing his AT every day.

(We are not really encouraging people not to practise their AT — but this instance of misplaced dependence needed to be addressed.)

Case 2 — John
John was an ambulance man who was experiencing increasing episodes of temper and aggressive feelings. He was becoming more and more withdrawn from his family and work colleagues. His teenage daughter caused him great frustration, and he found that he had to leave the house for hours on end to walk off his temper. He also suffered frequent bouts of Irritable Bowel Syndrome, with nausea, pain and diarrhoea. During the AT course, he was able to work through feelings of anger and grief brought about by the nature of his work. He also started to keep a journal, and to make use of the support systems offered through work. His mood quickly settled, his family relationships improved, and so did his IBS symptoms. He felt much better equipped to cope with situations and with his own feelings.

STRESS IN THE WORKPLACE
We see many cases where people have been put under unreasonable pressure by the expectations of their workplace.

Case 1 — Elinor
Elinor wanted to learn AT because of severe anxiety symptoms, low energy levels, disturbed sleep patterns, crying spells and frequent headaches. She felt permanently irritated by her family, and had little time for them. She had recently had seven weeks off work, where conditions had been extremely stressful for two years, despite numerous requests for help. Discussion about her work usually caused considerable distress. There was no discernible reason in her medical or social history to explain her current symptoms. (Issues around a previous un-satisfactory marriage had now been resolved, and she was in a supportive partnership.) Elinor attended group AT sessions, and her practice was most diligent. By the follow-up session, she reported that all her symptoms had greatly improved — she was almost free of anxiety and irritability; she was sleeping very much better, had hardly any headaches and was much less tearful. She reported having more time for herself and her family. Elinor went on to take her employer to court, fully con-fident that she could cope with this additional stress, and feeling strongly that her treatment at work should be brought to the attention of the public.

Respiratory Tract Disorders

Bronchial Asthma and Other Breathing Difficulties including: Hyperventilation; Chronic Bronchitis; Emphysema; Chronic Obstructive Airways Disease
Dr Luthe, when he first met Schultz and investigated AT, was most impressed with the way patients improved their asthma symptoms using AT. He wrote:

> The autogenic approach in the treatment of bronchial asthma is based on three factors: a) certain non-specific modifications of central nervous system activities ... b) localized organ-specific changes of a neuromuscular and circulatory nature,

and c) the patient's experience that he himself can deal effectively with the asthmatic attacks without the necessity for drugs.

Wolfgang Luthe, *Autogenic Therapy Vol. 2: Medical Applications*

We have seen the effects of the last point countless times. The client gains control over their condition — perceived as a huge breakthrough in gaining improvement.

Whatever the cause of any breathing difficulty, a strong psychological component tends to interfere, in the form of anxiety. If we cannot breathe comfortably, we fear that we will never be able to, and ultimately that we will stop altogether. This can interfere with any situation where the system needs to relax and 'let go', such as falling asleep.

Most sufferers of asthma say that the biggest problem with their condition is the fear that is engendered by it. AT seems to address this automatically. We often hear statements like:

- *My asthma is always worse when I am under pressure.*
- *When I feel angry, my asthma gets worse, but I can't seem to stop it.*
- *Stress always make my symptoms worse.*

Here, we need to acknowledge the underlying psychological contributory components of the disease. Suppressed emotions play a big part in asthma, and here all the Intentional Exercises have an important part to play.

As clients work through the Standard Exercise programme, they notice that their anxiety decreases. Also, their breathing feels easier before they even reach Standard Exercise 4, which includes the respiration formula. We, as therapists, may feel that caution is required in introducing this formula, but invariably the client is relieved to find a phrase 'just for me', and readily accepts its passive and trusting elements.

Case 1 — Beryl

Beryl, 69, had suffered from asthma for most of her adult life, and went through episodes of recurrent chronic bronchitis during her forties. She took three inhalers every morning, with the option to increase the doses if necessary ('but I prefer not to'). One was a steroid (cortisone derivative) to prevent inflammation building up and leading to a crisis; the second was for opening the air passages; the third was for relaxing the chest-wall muscles. She had been widowed, and was now living happily with a new partner (of ten years) who was eleven years older than her. Family circumstances had been difficult: issues with her elder son and daughter-in-law meant that she was losing touch with him and with her grandchild. When she started her AT course, these issues were paramount, and her first sessions were concerned with them.

Beryl reported a great deal of anger and distress, and yet her asthma was stable. She would normally have expected increased symptoms because of her distress, and the time of year ('My asthma is always worse in October because I'm allergic to mould spores'). She was sleeping well, on occasion sleeping through her alarm and forgetting to take her inhalers, with no ill effect during the day. By the end of the course, through her own understanding and changing perceptions, the relationship with her son had undergone a sea-change, and she realised that, because her own ego was feeling so much stronger, she had been able to let him go, and to grieve for the lost relationship. The use of Anger and Crying Exercises were enormously helpful in this. A spirometry reading during this time showed that her lung capacity had improved by 4 per cent. She was hopeful that soon she would be able to decrease the inhaler which 'opens' her bronchioles. She said: 'I am open — I know I am'.

In addition, Beryl noticed that she felt 'happier' in her life, and she rediscovered her sense of humour. (The rest of her group observed her increasing tendency to tease and provoke laughter during the sessions.) By the end of her nine weeks, she reported that she was consistently forgetting to take her inhalers, as her reminder had been the 'puffing and wheezing' she experienced after bed-making in the mornings, and this was vastly improved.

Case 2 — Matthew

Aged 41, Matthew perceived himself as having problems with his boss, and he also suffered from asthma, requiring regular use of an inhaler. He was particularly sensitive to petrol fumes. Three weeks into the course, he realised that his anxiety about his asthma had reduced, because he could leave the house and visit his next-door neighbour without checking that his inhaler was in his pocket. (Asthma was not his prime motive for learning AT.) The following week he had a car accident on the way to work — there were no injuries but his car was a write-off. He noticed that he coped with the distress of this far better than his wife, who was with him. Moreover, during the subsequent few weeks when he had to walk to work, he did not need his inhaler at all — he did not react to the traffic fumes around him as expected. In addition, he gained enough confidence to influence his working relationships, which increased his sense of being in control — both of his symptoms, and of his working life.

Hyperventilation

This is often described as when a person 'over-breathes', or is breathing in excess of the body's needs. This is a normal response to stress or excess feelings of fear. If the body needs to prepare for fight or flight, the breathing will change in order to accommodate the extra requirement for oxygen. It is only when circumstances for this reaction are inappropriate that this style of breathing is abnormal. Then, the intake of oxygen exceeds the output of carbon dioxide, which, if persistent, causes imbalance in the acidity of body fluids and the blood flow to the brain. It is often encountered as a secondary manifestation of anxiety, but there are many persistent symptoms resulting from it which can lead to misdiagnosis. These include:

- *Cardiac* palpitations; chest pain; angina
- *Neurological* dizziness; faintness; visual disturbance; migraine headaches; numbness; 'pins and needles' in limbs
- *Respiratory* shortness of breath; asthma; chest pain; sighing
- *Digestive tract* swallowing problems; 'air swallowing'; heartburn; burping
- *Muscular* cramps; fibrositis; tremors
- *Psychological* tensions; anxiety; feelings of 'unreality'; depersonalisation; hallucinations (rare)
- *General* weakness, exhaustion, lack of concentration; poor sleep; nightmares; emotional sweating.

Hyperventilation is a more common disorder than may at first be obvious, and the person may be completely unaware of the problem. The good thing about AT is that effective treatment does not necessarily depend on accurate diagnosis or the patient's acceptance of it. Often, once anxiety levels are reduced, and the breathing formula reached, a spontaneous improvement occurs.

Your therapist should be able to put your mind at rest about the normality of the process, and explain that your symptoms can be reversed.

Case 1 — Maria

This 72-year-old had enquired about AT several years before she came to learn it. She had been told that she was hyperventilating, and she asked several questions about the approach to breathing in AT. She decided to take her consultant's advice and go on a special 'Breathing Techniques' course. If that didn't work, she would sign up for AT. Later, Maria did come to learn AT, and she found that it helped her breathing more than she had expected. It enabled her to let go of her obsession with constant monitoring, and to leave breathing to be normalised

---

> by her automatic regulatory processes. As a result, her sleep improved, along with her self-confidence that she could influence her own destiny.

UPPER RESPIRATORY TRACT (URT)

We should mention here that many of our clients who come to learn AT for other reasons report that recurring URT symptoms improve markedly. These changes will be noticed after a relatively short time using AT and include:

- Losing a nervous cough
- Improvement in shortness of breath
- No longer suffering from recurring sinusitis or catarrh.

Here, we would draw attention to the probable need for work with the Intentional Crying Exercise to help relieve these symptoms. Also, the incidence of succumbing to colds, coughs, flu and other infection is greatly reduced, which would indicate the increased efficiency of the immune system.

SKIN DISORDERS

The distressing fact about any skin condition is that it is visible to the naked eye. Sufferers often perceive themselves to be 'unclean', and this causes great psychological distress which can get in the way of normal everyday life. And yet the skin can heal to such an extent that, after a short time, the problem might never have been there.

We, the authors, are both aware that skin irritation can be a sign of just that — irritation. When symptoms have developed to such an extent that thickening or raised patches of skin are evident, there is probably a significant amount of repressed anger. We recommend using the Intentional Exercises with any skin condition, to enhance the work of the autogenic process.

ACNE

Case 1 — Henry

Henry was 25 when he learned AT. Somehow the acne which everyone had told him was just the problem of teenage hormones, had never left him. He had taken low-grade antibiotics for more than a year, and this had caused other health problems. His perception of himself was so poor that he could not make eye contact with anyone he did not know well. Although he had a degree, he was in a low-paid and dull job. It turned out that his school years had been difficult — with hypercritical parents, and friends who teased him too much, his self-esteem had sunk to rock bottom. He learned AT individually. His symptoms began to diminish spontaneously, and he applied for and got a new job. He was much more confident, able to look in the mirror and see 'my face — not just my spots'.

ECZEMA

Case 1 — Paul

A dentist of 34, Paul suffered eczema on his hands, which manifested in a stress reaction cycle. He wore gloves, of course, but his tolerance to them was nil when his symptoms were bad, resulting in his being unable to work. During the AT course, his skin flared up again — causing severe pain and itching, and he had to take some days off work. He persisted with the Standard Exercises, and used the Intentional Verbalisation of Anger Exercise. His eczema cleared up, and remained clear, through to the end of the course. Paul knew that he felt calmer, was sleeping better, and generally coped with stress better. He regularly used AT during his lunch-times, and always in those irritating times when patients did not show up for their appointments.

Case 2 — Olive
Olive was 25, and had suffered from eczema, especially on her legs, since childhood. She had kept her legs covered all through her teens, and had been caused much distress and frustration. Her symptoms simply improved during her AT course.

PSORIASIS

This distressing condition consists of patches of scaly skin on any part of the body. At its worst, the skin can get very rough and thickened. Sufferers usually report feeling depressed and embarrassed about 'showers' of scales which can fall from the skin or the scalp.

Case 1 — Sally
At the age of 52, Sally arrived with her AT therapist, complaining that she had been struggling with psoriasis symptoms for the best part of thirty years. She had been treated by skin specialists, been to Lourdes, used oils and herbal remedies, taken saline baths and followed a stringent diet. All of this had had 'no effect whatever'. Sally's story continues in her own words:

> [The psoriasis] affected my legs from the ankles, and badly on the knees and thighs, and the rash continued over the whole trunk ...[with] isolated patches on my chest and shoulders. My arms were affected by spots with not more than an inch of clear skin between them and the elbows badly scaled. My face was clear, but scaling was present on my scalp, behind the ears and just above the hairline at the back, causing itching and a heavy fall of 'dandruff'.

After six weeks of AT, Sally's skin was 'almost totally clear', and remaining affected areas were much improved. Three months later, her scalp had completely cleared ('now able to wear black and navy blue'); she was sleeping much better; she had reduced stress; and she had gained confidence (noticed by both her partner and her employer). She described herself as previously having suffered from 'treatment fatigue' and having had very little faith that anything could help her. However, '...my more relaxed outlook, coupled with the dramatic improvement in my skin condition, has given me ... a hope and optimism I have not felt in many years. AT has made a huge difference to my life.'

PSORIATIC ARTHROPATHY

This rare condition is one manifestation of very severe psoriasis, with symptoms affecting the joints (arthritic swelling, pain and movement restriction), as famously depicted in Dennis Potter's play, *The Singing Detective*. At its most severe, long bouts of hospitalisation and steroid treatment are inevitable, perhaps, in time, leading to serious and permanent disability.

Case 1 — Joan

Joan was 32 when she came to learn AT as part of a stress management programme at her workplace. She was curious to see whether AT would help her symptoms. She was managing to keep reasonably well — coping with full-time work, and resorting to using steroids if necessary. Her main symptoms were the psoriasis (especially in her scalp — causing permanent 'dandruff'), and pain in her wrists, fingers and knees. In addition, of course, she had the distress of her disrupted life. After using AT for four months, she reported that her hospital consultant was most impressed by her general health improvement, which at that time showed an arrest of symptoms rather than an increase. She was able to reduce her steroid intake. Joan was most upset that her consultant took the credit for her improvement, knowing, as she did, that she herself had addressed a great deal of the emotional content of her condition.

Surgery and AT

We would always hope that the best place for AT in surgery is in preventing the need for it. Of course, this is not always possible, so the best we can suggest is to use AT pre- and post-operatively, to help cope with the anxiety and to help recovery.

Physical Aspects

Some people have found that an AT exercise plays the part of a 'pre-med', significantly reducing anxiety and physical tension. Post-operatively, AT will usually help with recovery from general anaesthetic, and will encourage muscle relaxation which will reduce the need for analgesic (pain relieving) drugs. AT is likely to reduce the possibility of post-operative complications such as deep-vein thrombosis, embolism or chest infection.

Case 1 — Julia

At the age of 37, Julia, a nurse, underwent a partial thyroidectomy for the removal of a lump. She was already well-versed and practised in AT, and was curious to see how using it would make this surgical experience differ from previous ones. Attached to a 'pre-med', she found AT exercises entirely pleasurable, and any anxiety she had disappeared. When she came round from the anaesthetic, she vomited, but felt quite at ease with throwing out (literally) the poison in her system. After the operation, she practised AT whenever she could, and found herself clearing her lungs by coughing during her exercises.

Psychological Aspects

Any surgical procedure, whether investigative or therapeutic, is an invasion of the body, and is remembered in the subconscious as a threatening and painful event. AT discharges will sometimes reflect this — for example, tightness or pulling at the operation site. Anxiety before surgery can affect the whole experience, from receiving the anaesthetic to eventual discharge from hospital, and convalescence, because the negative feelings will interfere with the healing process. Acknowledgement of this is important to help speed up recovery.

If a part of the body has been removed — for example, in the cases of hysterectomy, limb amputation, and mastectomy — a form of grieving for it is paramount. Using AT may bring feelings to the fore, either focusing on the loss, or on the life-threatening elements of the situation. Intentional Exercises are invaluable, especially the Crying Exercise, but these may have to be explained to hospital staff, so that you are allowed to continue with them!

CHAPTER 9

FURTHER APPLICATIONS OF AUTOGENIC THERAPY

AT AND SLEEP PROBLEMS

> So — you are lucky enough to sleep badly? This is very good. You can spend all night practising autogenic exercises. This will do you more good than going to sleep.
>
> Dr Wolfgang Luthe

Many clients coming to learn AT will be experiencing sleep problems. This may be the sole reason for learning AT or it may be just one of many problems brought about by excess stress.

The effects of poor sleep are many and varied, the most obvious ones being tiredness, drowsiness and fatigue, with lack of energy and mood swings contributing to general malaise and poor general functioning. People also complain of poor decision-making and decreased ability to concentrate.

Some people have difficulty getting to sleep. Others have difficulty staying asleep. Some wake in the middle of dreams; some wake for no reason at all, often at the same time each night; some wake feeling un-rested; some are woken by other things — baby needing attention, partner snoring, animals making demands. All of this can lead to a build-up of anxiety related to sleep — or the lack of it.

Autogenic Therapy offers many tools for the insomniac and, more importantly, may deal with the underlying cause. Most clients report improvement in the quality of sleep — some managing on less than in the past. Many cope much better with periods of wakefulness, and recover more rapidly from loss of sleep.

There is often an early indication of a change in sleep patterns when embarking on an AT course, usually for the better. Such an indication might be one of the following:

- Getting to sleep more quickly
- Feeling more refreshed after sleep
- Having more vivid dreams.

DURING AN AT COURSE

Some people will become aware of their own 'sleep debt' quite early on, noticing a need to cat-nap after an exercise, or yawning more than usual. This is quite normal, and should be encouraged while the system rights itself. Where there is a need to stay alert, using the simple sitting posture will help.

As the course proceeds, some students may experience temporary sleep disturbance as a result of emerging emotional material. There are several ways to manage these scenarios:

- Use the Intentional Exercises to deal with the material.
- Use the Dream Formula (see below).
- Use the short-stitch exercise to get to sleep, or to get back to sleep.

All autogenic therapists have seen extraordinarily fast turnarounds, sometimes for people with long-standing sleep problems. From pacing around at night, wide awake, and ironing at 3 a.m., regarding bed as a battleground in which to 'win' a few precious hours of sleep, a person starts to look forward to the safe haven of bed, where delicious sleep is just the other side of an autogenic exercise.

Simply using AT exercises in bed, before sleep, brings about a calming of the mind, often stopping the 'mind chatter' of the day. This helps the gentle transition from hyperactive consciousness to the sweet oblivion of sleep.

AT INTO SLEEP

There is one time in the day when you can practise autogenic exercises without closing — at night as you fall asleep. As the mind allows itself to calm down, the 'autogenic process' continues to function even after sleep ensues. The more practised you are, the faster you will respond to this nocturnal 'training'. Often, people report that there is no point in practising exercises at night, because sleep occurs so quickly — after using only the first autogenic phrase. We always recommend using it anyway: the purpose of a night-time exercise is to allow sleep to follow — completion of the exercise is not compulsory.

If you wake in the night, do an autogenic exercise. It may well send you back to sleep. If it doesn't, at least you are using the time profitably, and allowing the body and mind to enter a deeply relaxed state. If you are still sleep-deprived, you may find that you can restore your energy by doing an autogenic exercise early in the day.

There are various personal formulae related to sleep issues. These may be introduced if needed towards the end of the course (see Chapter 6). However, do not use them too early. Sleep disturbance at the beginning of your training may be part of your autogenic process, and should be passively observed, then accepted.

DREAMS

Dreaming is a normal and important process often inhibited by our attitude/anxiety. There are a thousand ways to interpret dreams, but the significance is not so much in the content of the dreams as in the fact that dreams happen at all. It is easy to become judgmental about dreams — we classify them as 'good', 'bad', or 'nightmares'. All dreams, whatever our perception of them, are 'good', simply because they are happening.

The brain reviews information it receives, and puts it into context with our previous experience as a necessary part of normal function. It chooses to do this symbolically while we are at rest, in deep sleep, so that the conscious mind does not interfere with the process. However, if the brain is attempting to 'deal with' anxiety, it will often produce a 'bad dream' or 'nightmare' in its attempt to process this anxiety. Sometimes this 'bad dream' is so powerful that we wake up in the middle, so the conclusion is never reached. The brain needs to make another attempt at off-loading this anxiety, so again we wake in the middle of the 'nightmare', and again the attempt is aborted. And so, here is the 'recurring nightmare' — it is a dream experienced as 'bad', and we try to escape from it by waking up.

Further, we may wake because unconsciously the brain is resisting a period of REM sleep, 'knowing' that a dream is on its way. We don't know why we have woken, but there may be difficulty getting back to sleep.

AT helps this dilemma in two ways. First, you may notice that your dreaming is spontaneously more vivid, in 'glorious technicolor', with strong themes, in the early stages of an autogenic process. Often this dies down again, and the person will report a generally improved sleep pattern.

If sleep is still disturbed after a few weeks, the person might begin to use a dream formula. This is a simple, positive phrase, used in evening/night exercises, which encourages the brain to develop a passive, receptive attitude towards dreaming. Nightly use of one of these phrases can change and improve a sleep pattern very quickly.

Examples of the Dream Formula

'*I passively accept the messages of my dreams.*'
'*I can go along with my dreams.*'
'*My dreams are interesting/enjoyable/therapeutic.*'
'*I love my dreams.*'
The formula is repeated three times, at the very end of each autogenic exercise, after 'I am at peace'. Use it only in afternoon and evening exercises, not morning ones.

CHILDREN AND DREAMS

Often children have recurring nightmares, sometimes so scary they are unable to speak about them. It is important never to dismiss the potency of these dreams by saying 'it's only a dream'. This can increase anxiety about them. Explain that dreams are sometimes scary, and they always happen when we are asleep so we are quite safe. These 'stories when we sleep' mean that we are making ourselves better as we face our fears in the dream and sleep through them.

Sleeplessness is very often related to anxiety. People who have undergone emotional traumas may well develop sleep problems, which seem completely unrelated to the original cause.

The person who seeks out their bed for ever longer hours of oblivion may be depressed, using sleep as an escape route. Or there may be a clinical reason for this need — anaemia, perhaps. In this case, AT will help the sleep, but do nothing for the fatigue, until the anaemia has been diagnosed and treated. Most insomniacs are aware if they feel 'ill'. They know the difference between clinical fatigue and poor sleep.

Case 1 — Linda
Linda, aged 35, had been badly injured in a head-on car crash two years before learning AT. She had been hospitalised for many months, had several episodes of surgery for multiple injuries, and had suffered nightmares and disturbed sleep ever since. As her brain attempted to resolve the trauma by reliving the accident, she would awake in a terrified cold sweat as the white van from the crash was in front of her nose. Early on in her autogenics course, she was given a dream formula to use, and she reported that her dream changed subtly, almost tricking her unconscious into 'staying with it'. The van became yellow rather than white; it whizzed past her right ear instead of getting 'stuck' in front of her nose. The dream no longer held its terrors, and her sleep and whole well-being improved.

Case 2 — Mary

Mary, who woke at 3.28 a.m. in the early hours of every morning, used the dream formula as a regular part of her AT exercises and found herself waking later and later in the mornings. She quickly dispensed with her fear of going to bed — recognising that she had been contributing to her own vicious circle of anxiety about the amount of sleep she was (not) getting.

Case 3 — Maurice

Maurice, in his fifties, had, for many years, had a disturbed pattern of sleep, which had worsened as a result of recent stressful changes at his work. In the first week of his course, practising short-stitch exercises only, he had slept through his morning alarm three times! Very brief exercises were all that he needed to restore his natural sleep patterns.

Case 4 — Jenny

Jenny was a single mother in her thirties, caring for her 11-year-old child who had learning disabilities, and her widowed mother. She had had disturbed nights ever since her son's birth. Following a bereavement, her symptoms had worsened, and Jenny was finding it increasingly difficult to cope. Her sleep started to improve initially, although in the middle of the course it worsened again when emotional material began to emerge, indicating the need for work with the Intentional Off-loading Exercises. There followed a week when she felt a constant need to sleep. Then things improved rapidly — sleep came easily, and its quality improved. Jenny was able to cope with her mother's deteriorating health, and felt able to face the future with the confidence of her new skills.

Case 5 — Liz

Liz, aged 32, happily married to her second husband, and with an 18-month old baby, came to learn AT to deal with insomnia. She described going to bed as 'like going into armed combat'. She needed the props of radio, thermos of drinks, clock (must count the hours), rituals and piles of books. She said, 'Why do I have this problem now, when life is treating me so well? Seven years ago I was desperately unhappy, coping with a terrible marriage, then a messy divorce, and I slept fine, held everything together (even my job) through it all. Now I have everything I could wish for, life is good, and I have a stress symptom I can't deal with.'

In time, Liz came to understand that the remarkable adaptation of the human being was the culprit of her circumstance. While she was going through her difficult divorce, she had to hold on, keep everything together, keep control of her life, and not break down under the strain. At the time, this stood her in good stead — she got through, she survived.

When she married again, life settled down, and she had a longed-for baby. Suddenly her symptoms of stress appeared in the form of insomnia. It was as though her mind was saying, 'Thank goodness I can now let go and deal with my unfinished business. I have been holding on to all that angst for years — now all is well, survival is assured, I can pay attention to the past and allow it to resolve itself.'

Liz used autogenic exercises and Intentional Off-loading Exercises. She understood the aspects of grieving for her first marriage, and gradually her sleep pattern improved. Soon she needed none of her props — she looked forward to going to bed, her last AT exercise being the best of the day. She no longer cared if, or for how long, she slept or lay awake. She had trusted her wise inner self to lead her through her process, and heal her system.

AT IN THE WORKPLACE

Both authors have experience of working in a variety of industrial settings. The benefits to a workplace of this type of self-development course are many. They include improvements in:

- Creativity
- Concentration
- Interpersonal relationships
- Health
- Morale
- Decision-making
- Motivation.

It is not necessary for *all* working staff to learn AT (although it helps). There is often a ripple effect: those close to the AT client can benefit too! Our clients have also found AT techniques invaluable for coping with interviews, and especially helpful when giving presentations, and in other public speaking. There is also useful application of AT in redundancy to help people deal with the emotional distress of losing a job, and the stresses involved in finding a new one.

We should not ignore that many health problems improve as well. Just because you learn AT at work doesn't mean that its effects are limited to work issues.

Case 1 — Brian
Brian joined a group of colleagues to learn AT. It was apparent that he did not get on with his colleagues, and his reputation was that of the office tyrant. He started the course with little enthusiasm — his motivation came from being told by his manager that if he didn't do something about his aggressive manner, he would lose his job. He found immediate benefits in improved sleep, and then became enthusiastic about his practice. At his follow-up session, he reported feeling a lot more laid back. He was enjoying his work, and his colleagues reported that he was a much nicer person who was getting on well with his staff, delegating more, and motivating them to develop themselves.

In an industrial setting, no one likes to admit that they are under stress at work. However, when they join an AT course there is no need to divulge the reasons for being there.

Case 2 — Clive

Clive joined a group of colleagues from a large company which offered AT as a personal development course. At the initial confidential assessment he revealed that he was suffering from sleep problems and was finding it hard to switch off when he got home from work. He found that he was bottling up a lot of frustration about his work colleagues. By the end of the course, he reported feeling a lot better about himself, and a lot more tolerant of others; he felt more in touch with his emotions, and was able to see his own faults more clearly. He found the Intentional Anger Off-loading Exercise useful as it helped him to deal with negative feelings, which resulted in his not carrying his resentment around. This improved the quality of his autogenic standard exercises.

Case 3 — David

David had recently been promoted to a management post which involved meeting prospective clients at social events. He got so nervous in these situations that he could not remember people's names or what they had talked about. Following an AT course, he was able to be much more at ease in social situations and, with the personal formula, 'names are interesting', was able to focus more on the clients and recall their details later.

Case 4 — Lisa

While her husband retrained for a new career, Lisa, at 35, was the main wage-earner, juggling a full-time career with a young family, having been promoted to a management position in a big company. She was aware of a lot of stress in her life, and headaches and fatigue were wearing her down. In addition, there were significant personality differences between her and her boss, and Lisa found herself taking time off sick with petty symptoms, feeling unable to overcome these.

Lisa's AT course was relatively uneventful, apart from the struggle in trying to fit AT exercises into her crowded schedule.

At first, she relied on the weekly session at work in which to do them. Then she realised that she would have to apply herself if she was to succeed in making the changes she wanted. She discovered how to use her train journeys for two daily exercises, and fitted in the third after she had read a bed-time story to her children. By the end of the course, her headaches had disappeared, she was sleeping well, and she had developed such an improved relationship with her boss that he came on the next AT course! She began to understand what her colleagues described as 'Managing Upwards' (keep the boss happy and kick your team), and decided that she would have none of it. Her management skills were open and honest, and she was instrumental in keeping AT going at her company for some years.

Case 5 — Margaret

Margaret, married for the second time and with a 13-year-old daughter, was three months pregnant when she came to learn AT. Her life was very busy, and she found it hard to find time to practise. AT before sleep became her lifeline, and some time later, after her baby was born and she was back at work, she realised how much she had gained from the original course, despite 'only paying it lip-service at the time'. She compared herself as a new mother after the big gap, with the previous time, and realised that her changed attitudes were about not only her own maturity, but also her increased tolerance to her teenage daughter, her husband and her colleagues.

Case 6 — Ron

Working as a maintenance technician, Ron did long hours and shift-work. This meant that for some AT sessions he had to come in while working nights. His therapist was willing to accommodate his shift work, but he recognised the value of the group support during the course, and chose this way. At the end of it, he was worried that he was feeling so laid back that he might lose his job! Closer questioning revealed that when he had to wait for spare parts, he could move on to the next task without anxiety. Before, he would have got agitated and tried to hurry things up. Now, he let it go, since there was nothing else he could do about it. So, he actually improved his performance at work — concentrating on the job in hand, and allowing others the responsibility to do theirs.

The workforce is often unfairly blamed for 'stress', when other factors should be acknowledged and dealt with. The employer who encourages his/her staff to learn AT, whatever the perceived origin of the stress, is using an enlightened approach in caring for their whole well-being. The effect of AT can be to increase performance − this is as beneficial to the employer as to the employee.

AT IN EDUCATION

There are many applications of AT in education for both the student and the teacher.

CHILDREN

During the 1970s, AT was introduced to schoolchildren in Canada, taught by specially trained teachers. At first, the focus was physical illness or problems such as stuttering or bed-wetting. Then other improvements became evident, such as improvement in sleep and eating habits, less irritability and fewer tears, and children appeared to get on better with their peers and with adults; school results improved, and teachers reported an improvement in attention, behaviour and participation (Luthe, Vol. III).

Case 1 — Robin
Aged 14, Robin was on the point of exclusion from his school. His behaviour was disruptive, his concentration span was woefully limited, and he was caught up with his peers in a cycle of

not caring. His parents did their best, but they all lived in a deprived area, which probably contributed to Robin's general feelings of low self-esteem. He was referred to an educational psychologist, who took Robin through a shortened AT programme. His attitude and behaviour improved dramatically, along with his ability to concentrate, and he avoided exclusion. His personal formula was: 'School is cool — I'm no fool'. (Robin learned AT individually — his AT sessions were very special, and, coming from a big family, he appreciated the attention.)

Case 2 — Peter

Aged 12, Peter had had a great many health problems, which were eventually seen as the manifestation of a school phobia. He had some learning difficulties, and although he was eager to work and do well, the struggles were enormous. For four years he had barely been able to complete a whole week at school, because of his symptoms. With very low self-esteem, Peter was in despair, as was his family. He did a shortened course of AT, using Standard Exercises 1, 2, 4 and 6. From the first week he seemed much more confident, able to maintain eye contact with his therapist. For the first four weeks of the course he attended school every day, with no ill effects. He looked bright, and he walked tall. Then he got an ordinary cold and sore throat, which were not the same as his normal symptoms. His mother learned AT as additional support for him.

Case 3 — Jason

Jason was a bright 13-year-old who suffered from migraine attacks associated with extreme anxiety about schoolwork. He was missing a lot of school as he would wake up suffering a migraine. These usually wore off as the day went on. He was doing schoolwork at home whenever the migraine would allow, but was still very worried about falling behind. He was taught modified AT, and given instruction in the Intentional Off-loading Exercises. He was enthusiastic about having his special exercises. His migraine attacks receded, he became less anxious about his work, and he used the neutralising formula 'Schoolwork doesn't matter'. He also found that he was able to spend more time on non-school activities.

Case 4 — Rosalind

Aged 11, Rosalind was a very poor sleeper. Her mother was concerned, as this was affecting her schoolwork and the rest of the family as well. After visiting the autogenic therapist, Rosalind decided against learning AT, but her mother, who had been encouraged to join her daughter, decided to go ahead herself. As a result, Rosalind's sleep pattern improved!

TEACHERS

A great many teachers come through our doors to learn AT. Often the catalyst is the stress experienced before an impending school and education inspection (in the UK this is known as an Ofsted report), or 'post-Ofsted stress'. Changes in the teaching profession are ever harder to keep up with, and with the stress of increased administration, and the changing influences in society, we regularly see many problems. These include:

- Overwhelming stress (which is often the cause of long-term sick leave)
- Low morale and self-esteem
- Frustration and anger
- Sleep problems
- Severe anxiety
- Migraine and headaches
- Low coping ability
- Exhaustion.

Case 1 — John

As a young teacher, John came to learn AT, suffering severe anxiety and panic attacks. He had had several periods off work and had been taking beta-blockers which he was trying unsuccessfully to manage without. He was disillusioned with teaching and was considering a change of career. He was enthusiastic about AT and had high hopes of curing his panic attacks. From the first week, he reported sleeping better and having vivid dreams (nature's way of dealing with anxiety). After some initial resistance, he used the Intentional Exercises with enthusiasm. At the end of the course, John reported that he was a different person. He had not had a panic attack since the third week of the course, and was enjoying his work much more. He had even applied for a deputy head post — confident that with his AT tool-kit he could deal with the stress involved.

Case 2 — Peter

Peter was a deputy head of a primary school facing an Ofsted inspection. He was the lynch-pin at work, because his school's head teacher was new, and the school was only just recovering from a serious fire. He was desperately overworked, and felt that he was functioning under par because of the intensity of his anxiety. His therapist was concerned that he might not pay proper attention to his AT simply because of time. But he did — determined to do something about his situation. Within a few weeks, he said that he no longer cared so much about the Ofsted inspection — he could only do his best. Suffice it to say that the school passed with flying colours, and Peter was anxiety-free. He had made very good use of his Intentional Off-loading Exercises, and felt more in tune with himself.

AT helps teachers to cope better and it can renew their enthusiasm for their work. Some teachers have gone on to train as autogenic therapists and now teach colleagues, parents and students.

Autogenic Therapy

Some Quotes from Teachers who Have Learned AT

- *The process and the discussions involved in the AT training enabled me to prioritise and rationalise issues to cope with the forthcoming Ofsted inspection.*
- *I lose my temper less and am more at ease with pupils. Less tired. Use humour more in class.*
- *AT gains in effect the more I do it.*
- *I think more clearly and lessen the feelings of being wound up.*
- *Gives me a moment to focus on myself.*
- *Blood pressure back to within normal limits. Migraines decreased in frequency but not gone completely.*
- *AT seems to give me a quick pick-me-up when I'm flagging.*
- *As a special-needs teacher, I find myself able to stand back from too much emotional involvement with the children's social issues, and give more to those areas I can influence.*
- *AT calms me down — I don't make impulsive decisions or react immediately to stressful situations.*

AT IN SPORT

There are many examples of the use of AT in sport, including some years ago, the Olympic pistol-shooting team. People involved in competitive cycling, golf, athletics, tennis, equestrian sports, archery, and team sports such as baseball, have all used AT to improve their performance.

AT can help to maximise potential in sport, by clearing emotional blocks, particularly performance anxiety, helping with motivation to train, maintaining a positive mental attitude, and improving concentration, co-ordination and focus. It also helps to prevent injury, caused by competing with tense muscles; and it helps to speed up recovery time after injury.

We often get positive comments from amateur golfers whose game has improved even though they came to learn AT for a quite different reason.

Case 1 — Peter

A keen golfer, Peter attended an AT course suffering from Irritable Bowel Syndrome (IBS). Following the course, he found to his surprise that, as well as a significant improvement in his IBS, his golf performance was also much improved. He was using the neck and shoulders partial exercise before hitting the ball, and this had helped his accuracy greatly.

Case 2 — Nick

Aged 42, Nick had come to learn AT to help his stress at work. However, during the course he let slip that he enjoyed clay-pigeon shooting, competing at national level. He found that his aim became more accurate, and he retained an attitude of calm throughout contests, which helped his concentration. He put the neck and shoulders partial exercise to good use during competitions, often in the moments between shots. This helped him to let go of what had gone before — he could stop himself dwelling on a previous poor shot, devoting 'full-on' concentration to the next.

A sportsperson needs to learn the optimum placing of an autogenic exercise in relation to their performance. The residue of the feelings of deep relaxation need to be cleared before good active concentration is at its best.

Case 3 — Paula

In her fifties, Paula spent her life running her stables, breeding and training horses. One day, half an hour after doing an AT exercise, she went to the training school to help with a particularly difficult young horse — breaking in this extremely nervous animal had been a great problem for all her staff. On this day, though, he responded well to her — and she ended up able to saddle him, and then ride him. Paula was convinced that her AT exercise had influenced the situation. So, a few days later, she did another exercise before taking a different horse around a

---

jumping circuit. And this was 'a disaster'. The horse simply went its own way, refusing to respond to her commands. After the ride, Paula reported that she wasn't at all surprised: she had felt herself to be too 'spaced out' to ride with good concentration. It turned out that the AT exercise was too close to the event, and the horse was affected by her 'post-AT' distraction.

Case 4 — Doreen

In her youth, Doreen had been a good tennis player, but lack of practice in later years meant that her command of the game had slackened off somewhat. One day, during a game with friends, she decided to use the neck and shoulders partial exercise between points, to help her serve. It was so successful that her opponent commented. 'What were you doing? You looked so concentrated before you served, I felt quite frightened!' Doreen won the match.

Case 5 — Steve

A sergeant in the army, Steve had been wounded in action some ten years prior to his learning AT. He led a pistol-shooting team and wanted to improve his concentration. He was surprised by the therapeutic aspects of AT, but gained a great deal from them — off-loading some of his trauma load acquired during his active service. The pay-off was that he began to win all his pistol competitions. His team-mates began to remark, 'What are you on?' as they watched him hit bull's-eye targets time and again. He said nothing to them — wanting to keep the secret to himself! To his therapist he explained: 'When I'm shooting I am really relaxed. Between shots we have to lower the arm, then raise it again to aim for the next shot. There is a time limit for doing this and I used to rush it and get flustered. Now I use "Neck and Shoulders" as I lower my arm, and I feel there is all the time in the world. Also, my concentration is "full on". I can think about that moment very intensely, and I am not distracted by other shots by my team or anything else.'

The personal and motivational formulae are extremely useful in any performance-related situation. Choosing these will depend on the hoped-for outcome, and what is needed to achieve it. For example, for the tennis-player:

- *My serve is strong and accurate.*
- *My racquet reaches every shot.*
- *I am strong and concentrated.*
- *I love tennis — I love playing my best.*

A runner used '*My legs are strong and untiring*' when he felt his energy beginning to flag — he could carry on.

These personal formulae always focus on you and your performance, and affect your performance. This is all we can influence. There is no point in 'attacking the other guy' — he is beyond our influence.

MENTAL REHEARSAL

The autogenic state can be used to carry out mental rehearsal for particular situations. As long there is no serious off-loading going on, and passive concentration is good, the altered state of awareness at the end of an exercise is an excellent place to rehearse the skills you need. Actors might 'go over' their lines and stage moves in this state; tennis-players imagine themselves performing their 'strong and accurate serve'; footballers can imagine all the muscles and eye-coordination they have to use in order to take the penalty shot.

When using mental rehearsal in AT, allow a minute or two to imagine the scene: the feel of yourself in your clothes, the floorboards under your feet, the sound of the crowds (whether cheering or boo-ing), the feel of the sun on your face, the warmth of the applause in the concert hall etc. These steps are important – helping to create the environment of the actual expected performance.

The advantage of mental rehearsal is that you never miss! The more your brain is given the opportunity to perform the task correctly in imagination, the more likely it is to happen in reality.

AT AND THE PERFORMING ARTS

Many therapists report stories of the positive effects of AT for actors, singers and dancers. Any of these activities involves rigorous training, along with extremely concentrated efforts when performing. Often the first task with AT is to off-load the tensions and frustrations associated with striving to be the best. Coupled with these issues is the stress of living the performer's life — the uncertainty of employment, living up to expectations ('You are only as good as your last performance').

The ability to switch quickly into the autogenic state helps to redress the imbalance of constant late-night 'wind-down' — often a problem after theatre or concert performance. It may or may not help performance nerves — most performers recognise that these are necessary to keep concentration at its best. However, where 'nerves' are too prominent (for example, the musician's hands sweat too much which affects their playing), AT can help to reduce this enough to make a big difference.

Mental rehearsal (see above) will also help. In a deeply relaxed state, the muscles can retrain to enhance their performance in reality.

Tension in the performing effort can impede the result: seeking to do our best can cloud the artistic creativity. The differences in the brain hemisphere functions are at work here. Intensive training (left brain) allows the processes of knowledge to assimilate in the whole body — the muscles used for the task, the alert senses (hearing, vision, touch). Perhaps the final stage is the performance itself, where creativity (right brain) and instinct can confidently link in with the technical/intellectual prowess.

Case 1 — Suzanne

A semi-professional singer for many years, Suzanne came to learn AT for other stress-related reasons. As an unexpected bonus, she found her singing greatly improved. She became less anxious about good performance, allowing herself to be good enough. 'The result meant that rather than over-breathing

---

and pushing the sound, I could relax, and allow and enjoy a much easier and better-quality performance. I used the neck and shoulder partial exercise while awaiting my cue.'

Case 2 — Iain

An actor and drama teacher, Iain came to learn AT to 'sort out my life'. He was caught in a spiral of anxiety about his work, which then led him to turn to alcohol, which caused difficulties in his marriage. By the end of his course, he found that he had almost eliminated his anxiety — several performances he was involved in had run smoothly with much less 'angst' than usual, and he reported, 'I have fallen in love with my wife again — we have both given up drink.'

AT AND DANCE

Clover Roope is a British Autogenic Society therapist who had a long career with the Royal Ballet, and is still teaching — using the Martha Graham technique.

She writes:

When I learned AT for myself I thought: 'If only I had known about this when I was still performing as a dancer.' The next thought was: 'If only I had had this skill before — when I was a student of dance in a professional school from the age of nine.' I felt saddened by these thoughts — the national training was, of necessity, extremely tough. AT would have steered me through minefields of physical, mental and emotional traumas, and I am sure my professional and personal journey through life would have been smoother.

Several mature dancers and dance teachers have learned AT … they are unanimous in concluding that the benefits of AT are far-reaching. They all commented first on their increase in confidence and self-esteem. This enables them to deal with relationship difficulties, and particularly with anger, which has probably been suppressed for a life-time.

This, along with positive outcomes in different physical symptoms, has profoundly affected their work situations, especially in their relationships with their students.

Case 1 — Ruth

A teacher of dance, Ruth was suffering quite severe anxiety, knowing how much students' futures were at stake when she was involved with major adjudicating and auditioning situations, sometimes in foreign countries with inevitable language differences. Ruth's autogenic process led her through her own past issues of anger and performance, and she found the Intentional Off-loading Exercises invaluable. Now she is aware how much AT helps her in all her professional situations: 'I know I can't do without it.'

AT AND RELATIONSHIPS

In any close personal relationship, when either partner is under stress, it will put a strain on both parties. If both partners are under stress, it is often difficult to find the time and the energy to work through problems. Assumptions might be made about feelings and attitudes, which causes serious misunderstandings. Inappropriate anger often leads to rows and tense arguments, when the underlying feelings might be hurt, loss, fear, anxiety or frustration. Unconsidered words are said that are hard to retract, and it is very easy for a downward spiral to develop.

Relationship problems are not often the main reason for doing AT, but they are a common component of a stressful life. We have witnessed remarkable turnabouts in relationships when only one partner has learnt AT. We often observe that learning AT 'can make or break a marriage'. By this we mean that when a partnership is in trouble, if one partner is able to face their feelings and doubts with honesty, the chances are that they will find a way to change the interaction with their partner. If the situation has gone too far, and separation is inevitable, but no action is being taken, AT may help the person to deal with the stress and emotion involved, and to move on with their life, finding the courage to make it happen. In other words, AT will usually help to mend a relationship which is OK underneath, but it won't remedy the impossible.

Case 1 — Julie

Julie came to learn AT because she was having sleep problems; she also complained of frequent headaches, and increasing anxiety. On assessment, she discussed her deteriorating relationship with her husband. He was in a stressful job and they were having frequent arguments. This left them both short-tempered with their two children, and family life was difficult.

Early in her AT course, Julia reported sleeping better. With more energy, she was able to give the children more patient attention. As the course progressed, Julia found that she was increasingly able to talk to her husband about potential problems, without it degenerating into a row. She was able to negotiate time for herself and, in return, agreed to her husband having time to play golf. Things in the family improved, and before the follow-up session the whole family enjoyed a holiday together.

At the follow-up, Julie reported feeling more 'laid back' about things — she felt happy to express herself with confidence and to ask for what she wanted. She was able to say 'no' to people, so she was no longer taking on things for school and work that she could not cope with. She realised that she had had no headaches since the early weeks of the course.

Case 2 — Jeremy and Sarah

When Sarah came to learn AT, she stated that she was about to leave Jeremy for another man with whom she had been having an affair. She was tired of always coping with young children and a busy social life, alongside Jeremy's demanding job. Sarah felt that there was no spark left in her marriage. She gained a lot from the course: improved sleep, reduced anxiety, more confidence and patience. She was hoping to get help in telling

Jeremy of her decision, and it became clear that she was terri-fied — not at all certain how he would react, and very afraid of his anger. A discussion developed into a useful awareness that, however much she might wish to, Sarah was not going to be able to protect Jeremy from his feelings. Once he knew, Jeremy's reaction was his, and Sarah had to leave him with it.

A few weeks later, Jeremy telephoned the therapist to book himself on an AT course! He and Sarah were still together, and the outcome of her confrontation with him had utterly sur-prised her. Far from being angry with her, Jeremy had been hurt and then very angry with himself. He had known that things were not good, but he had buried his head in the sand and was now kicking himself for it. Sarah realised that the spark was not out — it had just been buried for a while. She ended her affair, and together they worked on healing their relationship. A sig-nificant part of that was for Jeremy to learn AT to help his healing, and to unite them in looking towards the future.

Case 3 — Roger

Aged 48, a businessman with teenage children, Roger found that he had learned how to identify the triggers for trouble and prevent World War III breaking out at home! It was easier to take a step back.

CHAPTER 10

AUTOGENIC THERAPY: ORIGINS AND DEVELOPMENT TO THE PRESENT DAY

It was Dr Johannes Schultz (1884–1970), a neuro-psychiatrist, who originated the concepts of Autogenic Therapy. Together with Dr Oskar Vogt, he had spent many years studying the effect of hypnosis and deep relaxation on the mind and body. Both men were convinced that the workings of the brain were too complex and sophisticated to be totally satisfied by the new psychoanalytical methods of Freud.

Schultz first studied medicine (turning down an alternative career as a concert violinist), then broadened his outlook by studying psychology, philosophy, psychiatry and, finally, psycho-analysis. In the course of work in these other areas, he met Vogt, who became a major influence on his work.

During the 1920s, when Autogenic Training was beginning to be recognised and accepted in the medical world, Schultz met Freud. The following exchange was reported later by Schultz:

> Freud looked at me, sizing me up and said: 'Surely you do not believe that you could heal?' whereupon I replied: 'By no means, but I think that, like a gardener, I could remove obstacles hindering a person's true development.' 'Then we will understand each other,' answered Freud, ending our conversation with a charming smile.
>
> Dr Karl Wongstchowski, 'Schultz the Man', *British Association for Autogenic Training and Therapy Newsletter*, June 1987

Even though Schultz underwent his own training psychoanalysis, he was deeply intrigued with the mind–body link, and the influence played by emotions on the body. The term 'psychosomatic' was just beginning to be accepted as an explanation of how chronic physical (somatic) symptoms could have an emotional (psycho) origin.

In 1915, Schultz was appointed Professor of Psychiatry at Jena, moving to Berlin nine years later, where he worked not only in his own private practice but also, with Vogt, at the Kaiser Wilhelm Institute for Brain Research.

Between them, they developed their own approach to psychotherapy, embracing a psycho-physiological view. Vogt's previous work, on sleep and hypnotic states, and understanding 'somatopsychic' interrelations, was an extremely important influence on Schultz's later development of AT.

He and Vogt were concerned that Freud's psychoanalytic model did not serve the purpose of true healing as adequately as if the mind and body links studied by Vogt were also acknowledged.

THE PSYCHO-PROPHYLACTIC REST PERIOD

At the turn of the century, Vogt developed and refined this relaxation exercise as a method of treatment. These 'rest periods' were found, quite consistently, to reduce fatigue, and increase confidence and efficiency. Studies confirmed that the brain-activity changes which occur in sleep and hypnosis also appeared in these brief periods of deliberate relaxation exercise.

After an induction, when the therapist placed a hand on the patient's forehead, and the patient focused on the resultant warmth from the hand, the therapist verbalised the exercise. It consisted of repetitions of specific phrases which were designed according to the patient's condition, and were known as 'case-adapted'. Vogt encouraged his patients to continue practice at home — at first verbalising out loud for themselves, and then eventually allowing the phrases to be internalised as 'thought repetitions'.

There were certain elements in these procedures which Schultz used in his own work — namely, the preparatory discussion between patient and therapist; the step-by-step factual (structured) explanation of the treatment; and the choice of a suitably comfortable setting in which to practise the exercises.

These were the seeds of Schultz's Autogenic Therapy — they were sown shortly before the First World War.

Schultz wanted to produce a kind of hypnotic state without using the conventional hypnotic procedures. Vogt's hypnosis was induced without the invocation of heaviness and warmth — and yet more than 60 per cent of subjects reported feelings of heaviness and warmth during hypnotic induction. So, reasoned Schultz, why shouldn't we achieve the same state of relaxation by offering a suggestion of heaviness and warmth in the limbs?

To these he added a further ingredient — passive concentration. Repetition of the words (even as silent thought repetition) about heaviness and warmth in the limbs needed to be done in a casual, non-striving manner.

In time, Schultz realised that his patients could produce a self-induced shift of mind-state (later named the autogenic state). This resulted in a deep calmness — normally difficult, if not impossible, to produce at will.

THE AUTOGENIC DISCHARGE

As discussed in Chapter 2, the autogenic discharge is an important part of any autogenic process. But here Schultz and Vogt disagreed fundamentally, and it was many years (the early 1950s) before Vogt finally conceded that Schultz's view on this had been correct.

We now know that during autogenic exercises it is possible for the subject to maintain passive concentration on the thought-repetitions, while adopting the attitude of passive observer, casually noting and accepting responses. These responses are many and varied, and might consist of small muscle twitches, itching, fleeting discomforts such as headaches, palpitations. Or they might feel more extreme, such as a sudden need to cough, laugh, swallow or yawn, or 'gasp' a breath. There might also be emotional discharges — feelings of irritation, or watery eyes.

These discharges, or releases, as we now understand them, will occur during any kind of relaxation. However, Vogt regarded them as 'interferences' in the process, requiring that they should be suppressed, or the exercise stopped. For example, if a need to laugh was observed in one of Vogt's patients, he considered this to be a sign of hysteria, requiring immediate ending of the exercise. Schultz welcomed and encouraged these small transient changes, recognising them as indicators of a re-balancing process.

AUTOGENIC OR HYPNOTIC?

In the early days, Schultz described AT as a form of self-hypnosis. However, he was aware that some of the psycho-physiological changes occurring in AT were the opposite of those occurring in hypnosis.

The fundamental difference between the two is that AT is non-specific. The six Standard Autogenic Exercises are learned and practised in the same way by everyone. It is the diversity of response to them which creates the unique potential of AT.

While things have now changed somewhat, with modern understanding and methods, old styles of hypnosis were usually specific — the therapist engaged with the client in helping to deal with a particular problem. The therapist would induce the hypnotic state, and apply suggestions specifically designed to 'address' the problem. This approach is necessarily goal-oriented, and could be restricting. Also, there is an inherent likelihood that the client might develop a dependency on the therapist. This very dependency puts the therapist 'in authority' — the therapist knows best. In AT, the client retains their autonomy, the therapist playing the role of teacher, helper, facilitator, guide — the client is free to experience AT in any way that emerges for them.

Non-specific treatment — Autogenic Therapy — can bring about astonishing healing processes, unlimited by expectation, hope or authority.

Schultz believed that his patients/clients were the experts on themselves:

> Only he who lets himself be can be himself.
>
> Johannes Schultz

EXPANSION OF AUTOGENIC THERAPY

Schultz presented his findings about his new method to the Medical Society in Berlin, in 1926. In 1932, the first text on AT was published.

The use of AT was confined to Germany and Austria before and during the Second World War. Later, Schultz was joined in his research and development by Dr Wolfgang Luthe, who, after World War 2, emigrated to Canada, and was appointed Professor of Psycho-physiology at the University of Montreal. Invited by Professor Hans Selye to give autogenic courses at the new 'Institute of Stress', Luthe was acknowledged as one of the world's most outstanding specialists in the domain of stress research. Luthe introduced AT to Japan (where many studies have been done), and formed the International Committee for the Co-ordination of Clinical Application and Teaching of Autogenic Therapy.

Dr Luthe, by his own admission, was at first very sceptical about the claims he heard about AT. In the early 1930s, he was a young house doctor on a medical ward, when Schultz was invited to work with asthma patients, using AT. From being a hardened sceptic, Luthe was forced to change his view when he saw the results on his own ward. Medication was significantly reduced, or even eradicated. Moreover, he witnessed the psychological change in his patients, as they became empowered by the real possibility of influencing their own destiny in terms of their healing processes.

During the 1960s and 1970s, when the rest of the West was in the grip of 'Valium-mania', and gradually realising the dreadful harm of tranquilliser dependency, in Germany, a course of AT would be prescribed by GPs with increasing regularity and acceptance.

Schultz and Luthe collaborated on the first four volumes of the seminal texts about Autogenic Therapy, published in 1969. In the meantime, Luthe had developed an important extension to basic

AT: Autogenic Neutralisation (see Chapter 11). This work is published in Volumes 5 (1970) and 6 (1973).

AUTOGENIC THERAPY IS PSYCHOTHERAPY

While Luthe worked on his neutralisation process in Canada, Schultz in Germany was joined by Dr Klaus Thomas in developing the 'personal growth' dimension. AT had been shown to be effective in many psycho-physiological conditions, and attention was directed to the number/types of condition which AT might help.

Schultz had broadened out the Standard Exercises to include 'intentional formulae' (which were more akin to the specific post-hypnotic suggestion, with a desired 'goal') and the organ-specific formulae. They were incorporated within the context of the autogenic exercise, despite their specific content. In the UK and Ireland, these types of formulae are known as personal and motivational formulae (see Chapter 6). Dr Klaus Thomas has written several books (in German) on them.

MEDITATIVE EXERCISES

These were first developed by Schultz, then elaborated upon by Luthe and by Dr Klaus Thomas (see Chapter 11). They aim to facilitate the visual elaboration of phenomena occurring in the autogenic state. Dr Luthe was firmly of the opinion that these should not be used until the risk of further off-loading was minimal — that using autogenic meditative exercises too soon after learning basic AT could have a damaging effect.

DEVELOPMENTS BY DR LUTHE AND OTHERS

Luthe's experience in working with AT led to research which focused on the drop-out rate of some clients, possibly resulting from the time it took to work through the Schultz method. As described in Chapter 5, he developed the *Intentional Off-loading Exercises* as an invaluable addition to standard AT. The *short-stitch* and *partial exercises* contributed to the variations of pacing AT —

the standard course could be modified easily according to the client's reactions.

In addition to the modifications on Schultz's standard AT, Luthe extended the basic self-righting principles and devised the advanced methods of Autogenic Psychotherapy — *Autogenic Neutralisation* and *Creative Mobilisation Technique* (see Chapter 11).

The advanced methods of AT are used much less frequently than the standard level. Dr Klaus Thomas's 'Advanced AT' used Schultz's meditative exercises. Dr Luthe's 'Autogenic Neutralisation' is well-documented in Volumes 5 and 6 of the six-volume texts, but during the 1960s to 1980s he trained only a handful of medical therapists to use it. The British Autogenic Society aims to change this situation, as the few therapists using it in the UK and Ireland find it to be a fast, in-depth method of psychotherapy which gives power to the client.

Dr Heinrich Wallnöfer (University of Vienna) developed his Advanced Analytical Autogenic Therapy, in which the standard exercise is practised and the subject lingers in the 'state', allowing the mind freedom to roam and explore any arising images or thoughts. The initial stages of this always need the guidance of an experienced therapist. After the exercise, these effects are written down and examined/analysed by the subject. These analyses are discussed with the therapist at regular intervals.

All these refinements/developments are designed to facilitate the fundamental autogenic process of self-regulation, allowing the system to move towards homeostasis as quickly and as thoroughly as it can. With these variations of approach, therapists have at their finger-tips a comprehensive means of helping clients through their process, in spite of perceived difficulties (resistance) en route.

All of this counts for nothing, however, without the motivation of clients. If you want AT to help you to bring about change in your life, frequent practice and real engagement with the process is essential. As ever, we re-iterate the training element in Autogenic Therapy — the exercises will not 'do themselves'. With these extensions of basic AT, however, a wider approach and open-mindedness by the client to their processes is essential.

How Does Autogenic Therapy 'Work'?
What are the Processes Involved?

Several theories have been put forward in an attempt to explain exactly how AT 'works'. Three are recognised, and they all carry the strong possibility of truth. It may be the case that we will never know for certain exactly what the biochemical processes are that bring about such profound change in mind and body — seemingly without trying.

Figure 12: Left- and Right-Hemisphere Functions in the Brain

Left-Hemisphere Activity *Function predominates when active*	**Right-Hemisphere Activity** *Function predominates when passive*
Analytical thought	Instinctive thought
Scientific orientation	Intuition
Logical thought	Empathy
Concern with detail	Use of imagery; recognition of faces
Mathematical calculations	Creativity — appreciation of art and music
Speech and foreign languages	*Spatial* awareness
Rote learning	Process orientation
Striving for results — goal oriented	Lack of concern for results (goals) or performance
Worrying	Holistic thought
Social conditioning	Expression of feelings
Summary: Left-brain activity uses energy, and it is tiring to maintain this kind of concentration for long periods.	*Summary:* Right-brain activity allows physical relaxation, release of tension and recovery in mind and body. It is effortless, non-striving and refreshing — you replenish your energy.

1. NEUROLOGICAL MODEL

This is perhaps the most-used model because it can be backed up by research using EEG studies showing brain-wave activity in different states of consciousness. This simplistic view is probably the easiest to grasp in relation to explaining the mechanism of rebalancing.

In a normal alert state of consciousness the dominant left hemisphere takes priority over the less dominant right hemisphere.

When we look at the differences in functioning of the left and right hemispheres of the brain (Figure 12), we see how important each function is. There should be equality between the logical and learned processes (conditioning) of the left hemisphere, and the instinctive, spontaneous activity of the right brain. Information crosses the *corpus callosum* between the two hemispheres in a free, healthy exchange.

However, thanks to interference during development, the channel from the right brain to the left becomes distorted, resulting in information about, say, feelings, not 'getting through'. There may be a strong communication the other way, however, so that thoughts/commands, are imposed on the right hemisphere *from the left*, which inhibit its spontaneous activity.

Factors in Hemispheric Inhibition
Personality Development

In a perfect world, we might become a successfully integrated personality — dealing with our emotions and feelings, then making sense of them. We would function in a non-repressed mode, with full understanding and maturity. Unfortunately, this is highly unlikely in today's world. It is suggested that, as children, we learn to process traumatic disturbance by making a choice between the 'feeling' and 'thinking' modes, as using both modes can be too complex and overwhelming for the child. This means that the brain's processing is unbalanced, and biased towards the favoured way. As we grow older, attempts are made by the brain to integrate these forms of operating (perhaps causing psychosomatic symptoms).

Effects of Education

As the intellectual requirements of education encourage ever more use of the quick-thinking left hemisphere, the person becomes less able to connect with their feelings, perhaps judging them as unimportant, then dismissing them.

Traumatic Events

The normal mode of processing trauma is through dreaming or entering spontaneous meditative-type states which encourage the processing of the memories. However, if the level of material is too much, the brain will not be able to deal with it, and a kind of selective filter will seal off the right hemisphere with the memories within. Even similar memories (which might have helped recall of the original) are also hidden. This could explain the anomaly of what happens to memories of abuse in childhood.

The Emotions and Culture

We often learn from an early age that it is unacceptable to cry, to be angry or even to vomit, and we supress these feelings.

Then, hemispheric functioning becomes unbalanced, and this is usually in favour of the left (dominant) hemisphere. 'Dominant' is the appropriate word for its controlling, fast activity. As the instinctive activity of the right hemisphere is suppressed, feelings can be in-accessible: the 'right brain' seemingly under-used as the dominant 'left brain' takes over. In some cases, despite our Western culture, this position might be reversed. Here, AT can help the re-balancing of the dominant-right-brained person, helping to develop their logical skills and easing the scenario of too much feeling.

We aim to redress the balance with AT, and this is supported by evidence:

- Studies in brain-wave activity show changes commensurate with the altered state of consciousness of meditative states.
- Increased dreaming is reported — greater intensity and 'glorious technicolor'.

- Discharge activity (emotional and physical) brings about reduction in symptoms.
- There are reports of increased creativity and holistic awareness.

2. LUTHE'S GENETIC CONSTELLATION THEORY

This is a complicated theory which Luthe first put forward in 1983. It suggests that at any given point in our lives we may reach or recognise a possible three different concepts of the Self:

a) The Authentic Self
b) The Natural Self
c) The Artificial Self

If we were to take the concept of the 'Authentic Self' as a perfect 'being' at its conception, without distortion through any internal or external factors, it would be 'genetically concordant'. There would be a suggested limit of this person's potential, which leaves room for growth and development, always towards the potential limit — towards 'satisfaction'. Can this potential be realised, to enable that person to remain concordant with their authentic being?

The answer is: yes — as long as the person is given input and encouragement which is compatible with their potential. This will provide concordance. For example, if this person has musical or artistic talent, they have been encouraged to develop this. The likelihood is that they are at peace with themselves too. In this case, the *Natural Self* — that is, 'the person we are at any given moment in time' — is still in tune with the *Authentic Self*. This person is lucky.

Discordant, Disproportionate and Anti-Homeostatic Development

When there is too much pressure in areas where we have too little ability, the demand exceeds the resource. The areas of greatest potential have not been allowed to flourish and develop. In addition, this person has been forced to follow a path to which they are obviously unsuited. For example, the artist who is now an accountant — this person has not followed where their heart sings. They have developed their Natural Self to accommodate the discrepancies, but at what cost?

Interference with developing the potential reduces inner harmony, causing increased anxiety, insecurity and depression, reduced ability to adapt, and, ultimately, psychosomatic disease.

Artificial Self

The Natural Self is evenly developed, but it is *artificial*. This person has learned to adapt in an alien setting. They may not be consciously aware that all is not well. Perhaps issues of existentialism are around. (*'Is this all it is?' 'Is life simply about keeping up my mortgage and changing my car every two years?'*) Psychosomatic symptoms can appear here too.

Summary

The inherent potential in any individual can be severely distorted. It is possible that AT will help a person to reverse the effects of damaging experience and rediscover their Authentic Self. The aim of AT is to help the system to readjust. As self-awareness increases, the Natural Self of today begins to rediscover the original potential of the Authentic Self, as they recognise the Artificial Self. In time, the Artificial will reduce its potency, and the Natural Self will become more in tune with the Authentic Self.

3. THE HOMEOSTATIC THEORY

In 1981 a model of AT was proposed by Paine, Pensinger and Oliphant. This is an attempt to illustrate the concept of self-righting that we have come to take for granted in our teaching and experience of AT.

The theory is based on the assumption that our well-being, immunity and natural rhythms are explained in terms of the vibrational frequency of molecules. When stress disturbs these fundamental 'quantum frequencies', our positive health (homeostatic balance) is harmed. At the 'first line of coping', this damage is usually redressed by spontaneous dreaming or meditative-type activity. If AT is used at this stage, the self-righting process is greatly enhanced, through AT discharges.

If there is too much stress, and the system becomes overloaded, and the next line of coping is blocked, the effect may be the appearance of psychiatric symptoms, or functional disorders leading to decreased immunity (infections, cancer) or psychosomatic illness.

AT helps to redress the balance, allowing re-establishment of the fundamental quantum frequency.

AUTOGENIC THERAPY IN THE UK AND IRELAND

AT has been practised and taught in London for many years, quietly in the private practice of Dr Karl Wongstchowski. After an earlier career in orthodontics, he trained in psychoanalysis, and in AT with Dr Johannes Schultz. Dr Wongstchowski became an Honorary Member of the British Association for Autogenic Training and Therapy at its inception in 1984, and remained a supporter of our work until his death in 2000, at the age of 101.

During the 1950s and 1960s, AT was being used increasingly in Italy and France, but it seemed slow to move into Scandinavia or Britain. Even in the USSR, athletes and astronauts used AT to help their mental training for arduous tasks ahead.

Britain and Ireland seem to have been the last outposts in Europe to have 'caught on'. Bringing Mohammed to the mountain did not work: Schultz, Luthe and Thomas all came to lecture in Britain. Luthe remembered half of his audiences walking out of his lectures. Why?

Luthe's view was that the medical and psychological establishments did not at all like the idea of giving the patient their own autonomy. The premise of AT is that the client (patient) is in charge. The successful outcome of treatment does not depend on the interpretation of another person (therapist). The therapy is self-applied, and the process belongs to the client, not the therapist. Short-term, or brief, therapy used to be frowned upon, and, without first-hand knowledge and understanding of AT and its potential, it is not surprising that 'conventional' doctors and psychoanalysts did not approve of it.

In the mid-1970s, Dr Malcolm Carruthers (then a consultant clinical pathologist at the Maudsley Hospital), in the course of his research into heart disease, heard about AT, which was being used in Canada at the Stress Institute. At the time, new connections had been made between stress and the cardiovascular system, highlighting the debilitating effect the former has on the latter. Carruthers and his then wife, Vera Diamond, a psychotherapist, spent time with Dr Luthe, learning AT for themselves — the basics of Creativity Mobilisation Technique; and Vera was also trained in the use of Autogenic Neutralisation.

The autogenic movement grew in London, and further afield, with professional training courses designed for doctors, nurses, psychotherapists and counsellors. Luthe came over to co-lead the training courses which were held in 1982 and 1983, and gave his blessing to the British Association for Autogenic Training and Therapy, which was formed in 1984. The name changed in 1999, as a permanent headquarters was established at the Royal London Homoeopathic Hospital in London.

THE BRITISH AUTOGENIC SOCIETY

This is the professional and regulatory body for autogenic therapists in the UK and Ireland. It sets the educational standards for therapists, and acts as the information resource for therapists and the public. It also liaises with other autogenic societies around the world.

British Autogenic Society is a member of the UKCP (United Kingdom Council for Psychotherapy), EAP (European Association for Psychotherapy), and ICAT (International Committee for the Co-ordination and Clinical Application of Autogenic Training and Therapy).

BECOMING AN AT THERAPIST

Teaching AT is a very rewarding job. To the new autogenic therapist in training, it is a revelation to see how people flourish as they use AT for the first time. We have spoken throughout this book about the positive aspects when someone learns AT:

- Being enabled to fulfil their potential
- Experiencing the unfolding process of self-development
- Getting relief from pain and illness
- Learning to take care of themselves
- Developing tools for the rest of their lives
- Gaining a feeling of control over their lives.

Now we are recommending teaching AT as a truly remarkable and unique journey for us as therapists. When our clients say, 'Thank you', we have to reply, 'But you have done the work. You have kept at it, worked hard and discovered a lot — well done'. This gives us great job satisfaction.

CHAPTER 11

ADVANCED AUTOGENIC THERAPY

For most people, the basic Standard Exercises of Schultz's Autogenic Therapy stand on their own, requiring no further follow-up or development. Occasionally, it may be necessary to take people into further areas of exploration, using advanced methods of AT. This would be suggested for those who are curious as to how they might increase their self-knowledge, or for those who need to further their healing, through allowing deeper off-loading. We describe here three ways in which AT can be used for these purposes, although not all autogenic therapists offer these advanced methods. However, this book would not be complete without introducing them.

AUTOGENIC MEDITATIVE EXERCISES

After some months of practising Autogenic Standard Exercises (Schultz recommended six months to a year), the mind is able to switch easily into the autogenic state and can maintain that state for twenty to thirty minutes. There may be a growing experience of a completely neutral state within or at the end of an exercise. This is a period when no formula is running and there is no experience of time passing. Initially, you know that you have been in this state only when you come out of it. There may be an emerging awareness of colour or floating shapes.

These experiences are more likely to come about once the system has re-balanced and has no great need for Intentional Off-loading Exercises. The therapist will need to establish whether this is the case, because emerging emotional material could act as an intrusion and block the deeply neutral state needed for meditative exercises.

This is now an opportunity to train parts of the brain that offer some profound, and generally pleasant and insightful, experiences.

Schultz developed a set of seven exercises to enable people to access these upper levels and realise the further potential of the autogenic process. They are described in the first volume of *Autogenic Therapy* by Schultz and Luthe. These exercises are designed to develop an ability to produce mental images, which can then be manipulated and taken in a desired direction.

Meditative exercises are initiated with the aid of the therapist, with several weeks of practice at home between sessions.

Luthe describes the necessity to prepare the ground by ensuring that the mind–body system is cleared of any need to off-load, and training the subject to continue Standard Exercises for increased periods of time even when there are environmental disturbances. It is also necessary to be able to induce the autogenic state quickly and easily.

GROUP SESSIONS — HELD APPROXIMATELY ONCE A MONTH
Following instruction, the exercises are practised with very little intervention from the therapist (this can take thirty to forty minutes). Then, experiences are discussed when the exercise has finished.

FIRST MEDITATIVE EXERCISE —
SPONTANEOUS EXPERIENCE OF COLOURS
This involves a short induction into the autogenic state using brief formulae, usually heaviness and warmth in the limbs. There follows a period of passive focus on any visual phenomena which may emerge. These may at first be a vague impression of drifting grey shapes, general imagery or vague colours.

After some practice, perhaps of several weeks, a particular colour may begin to appear, which is individual and may be of personal significance. This will usually fill the visual field, and, with practice, the trainee will be able to gain access to this colour which they can with increasing ease identify as 'my colour'. It is important to let the same colour develop spontaneously without any striving or manipulation. It is not unusual for trainees to have experienced some of these visual phenomena during the standard AT training.

Case 1 — Marjorie

A 36-year-old neurologist, Marjorie, wrote: 'My mental field of vision became gradually filled with an intensive blue which showed tendencies toward red and purple tinting. It seemed as if I were living in blue-purple atmosphere, and this was accompanied by an extraordinary increase in sensations of warmth'.

(Example of Meditative Exercises from J.H. Schultz and W. Luthe, *Autogenic Therapy*, Vol. 1)

SECOND MEDITATIVE EXERCISE —
EXPERIENCE OF SELECTED COLOURS

After the brief AT induction, it is usual to start with the individual colour as developed in the previous exercise. During this, the therapist will suggest another colour — this may develop more easily if it is related to the individual colour, such as violet from blue, or orange from yellow. If a particular colour proves difficult, it may be linked to an object of that colour, such as green grass or blue sky.

The main focus, however, remains on the colour, the experience usually being of cloud-like formations, vapours or amorphous shapes. With a few weeks' practice, it becomes possible to work through a spectrum of colours. Most experiences of colour are deeply pleasant and calming. However, some colours may bring about uncomfortable feelings — this is recognised as being part of the self-regulatory process.

Case 2 — John

A 60-year-old man, John, had suffered insomnia for about twenty years. He had particular difficulty falling asleep. Various types of treatment had remained without satisfactory effect. The regular practice of the six Standard Exercises did not bring about any improvement. About four weeks after he had started practising visualisation of colours (First and Second Meditative Exercises) he noted more intensive effects during the Standard Exercises. Coinciding with this phase of the treatment, the patient started falling asleep without particular difficulty and enjoyed a good night's rest.

(Example of Meditative Exercises from J.H. Schultz and W. Luthe, *Autogenic Therapy*, Vol. 1)

THIRD MEDITATIVE EXERCISE — VISUALISATION OF OBJECTS

Beginning the same way as before, the trainee passively focuses on the spontaneous development of an object. This can take longer than colours, possibly forty to sixty minutes. At first, the image may be fuzzy or only part of an object may present itself, but with passive concentration it gradually becomes clearer. Once objects are readily and clearly evoked, the subject is ready to proceed to the next exercise.

Case 3 — Susan

'To start the exercise I was looking at a vase and feeling its shape and texture. I could visualise the vase, vaguely at first, and then it became more solid and vivid. I experienced it in three dimensions — really solid ....'

FOURTH MEDITATIVE EXERCISE — VISUALISATION OF ABSTRACT CONCEPTS

Here the trainee focuses on concepts such as 'justice', 'truth', 'freedom' or 'beauty'. A variety of individual experiences will be reported — some may 'see' the word, written or printed, or hear it repeated; some will be aware of a personal significance, others experience imagery of a film-like nature, sometimes expanding into surreal fantasy. Descriptions suggest that the trainee has entered a world beyond reality (sometimes using words such as 'like angels'). As with dreams, these are of a self-regulatory nature and can contain important symbolic information for the trainee.

Case 4 — Peter

The abstract concept: Freedom. 'At first I see a beautiful white horse breaking out of a corral. I hear the song: "Don't fence me in." I see the horse, disappearing in the distance, galloping. The mountain range appears with a lonely figure on top of one of the peaks. Then I see an orator speaking from a platform (freedom of speech). Then I see open doors (freedom of movement). Then marching soldiers (fighting for freedom). Then playing children (freedom of youth).'

(Example of Meditative Exercises from J.H. Schultz and W. Luthe, *Autogenic Therapy*, Vol. 1)

FIFTH MEDITATIVE EXERCISE —
EXPERIENCE OF A SELECTED STATE OF FEELING

After some weeks of meditating on the experience of abstract objects, the subject can begin to focus on a specific state of feeling. This may be a remembered feeling from the past, or the evocation of a desired feeling in particular circumstances. The experience is again varied, but often a film-like experience of the situation occurs, with accompanying feelings of well-being, such as that experienced when ascending a mountain to view the world or when standing by the sea, or walking in a pleasant garden. The focus is on the individual person — no other is involved.

Case 5 — Diane

'I am walking by the sea, then I walk into it and along the sea-bed, down and down into silent blue-green depths. There are objects from my life strewn across the sea-bed — things I have

---

> not thought about for years, and no longer have. I recognise them with pleasant nostalgia. I find a chest like an old pirates' treasure chest. I know I can open this and find new treasures. As I open the chest, a bright light envelops me and I enter an infinite space filled with light. The feeling is of extreme well-being — safe and secure.'

SIXTH MEDITATIVE EXERCISE —
VISUALISATION OF OTHER PERSONS

Now the subject of the meditation moves outwards from the self, to focus on other people. First, this is encouraged with a neutral person with whom we have no emotional ties — the postman or shopkeeper. Images of people with whom we have familial links are often more difficult to hold in the beginning, because they are strongly associated with positive or negative emotions. The images will become easier and more concrete with practice, the clarity of features being similar to that experienced during dreams. Eventually, it is possible to focus on more significant people, allowing clarifying insights and conclusions to be drawn about relationships and attitudes towards the other person.

Case 6 — Theresa

'For a few minutes I see the mailman. I think he is a pleasant man and wonder what kind of a life he leads. Does he realise the emotional implications connected with his job, being a carrier of good or bad news? How many people expect him in happy anticipation and how many are afraid of what he may bring? ... I see a former governess of mine who was with me when I was 9 to 11 years old. Later she went to Holland and came to see us when she was on home leave. Through her I met a Dutchman, who became my very good friend, and later my husband's as well. Then many old memories come up. I see my husband, my children ... I remember instances and situations of which I have not thought for a long time.'

(Example of Meditative Exercises from J.H. Schultz and W. Luthe, *Autogenic Therapy*, Vol. 1)

SEVENTH MEDITATIVE EXERCISE —
ANSWERS FROM THE UNCONSCIOUS

The last meditative exercise uses passive concentration to focus on questions to the subconscious: '*What do I want?*' '*What do I feel about my work?*' '*Who am I?*' '*How can I gain most out of life?*' The response to these existential issues will of course vary, and there may be film-like imagery that offers an opportunity to reflect upon and gain insight into the emerging feelings.

Case 7 — Maureen

'After about five minutes I see myself as a little girl of pre-school age playing in a sand-pile. I know that this is in a place where I spent my vacations with my mother and another woman and her little girl. Now, I am all alone. The thought strikes me that everybody is alone. Then I see before me a snapshot which shows me together with my mother. Then I see my father on his deathbed. Then I see Christ nailed to the cross. Then I see a former friend of whom I have not heard for many years. All these pictures follow each other in short succession, each taking the place of the preceding one without inter-mingling. I wonder what these people have in common and why they appear, seemingly in a connection. I think they were seeking "truth" and the knowledge of what life really is. That is exactly what I am trying to find out too.'

(Example of Meditative Exercises from J.H. Schultz and W. Luthe, *Autogenic Therapy*, Vol. 1)

In Germany, Schultz's Autogenic Meditative Exercises have been further developed by Dr Klaus Thomas and Dr Wallnöfer. The topics are similar, and we give a very brief overview here. In the UK, Tamara Callea runs courses in London using the German form.

SCHULTZ'S EXERCISES

- Evocation of colours.
  First one's own colour, then a list of six colours on demand.
- Contemplation of concrete objects
  Outer observation and then inner contemplation of objects chosen for their aesthetic value or sentimental value.
- Contemplation of abstract objects or values
  Themes are explored like 'justice', 'happiness', 'truth' and so on.
- Self-evaluation and view of humanity
  Who am I? What am I doing wrong? What is my path?
- Answers from the unconscious to existential questions
  Is being physically ill the worst thing? The meaning of work? What is better: happiness or justice? Living alone or in community? My image of death? Eternity? Immortality? The meaning of life? What are my characteristics and qualities? What do I really want? How do I wish to change? Am I good? What are others saying?
- Personality formulae, existential values, motivational formulae.

NB: Sensitive and deep material can be mobilised here and, therefore, the groups should be small (5–10 maximum). The trainer needs to be medically and psychologically trained to deal with the material adequately.

KLAUS THOMAS'S GUIDELINES
Weekly or fortnightly meetings, starting with a reduced version of the Standard Exercises.

- Spontaneous evocation of colour; evocation of specific colours
- Contemplation of concrete objects
- Contemplation of abstract objects: positive inner values
- Character building
- Journey to the depths of the ocean
- Journey to the top of the mountain
- Contemplation of spontaneous or selected themes.

THE POTENTIAL FOR AUTO-ANALYSIS

Wallnöfer suggests the potential for auto-analysis (as does Schultz).

These exercises are introduced one year after basic AT. The exercises are first practised in a group setting, then at home for at least two half-hour sessions during the week, then clients report back at the next group session.

The facilitator (therapist) avoids interpretations by either him/ herself or by the group members. A '*carte blanche*' attitude is encouraged (Luthe), and each group member is guided towards their own interpretation.

Wallnöfer's structure includes all Schultz's original meditative exercises, as well as the following:

- Geometric shapes developing before the inner eye
- Asking the unconscious (after about eighteen weeks)
- I am seeing myself (after about six months).

AUTOGENIC NEUTRALISATION

Dr Wolfgang Luthe developed this extended method of Autogenic Therapy during the 1960s and 1970s. His books on the subject (*Autogenic Therapy*, Volumes 5 and 6) were published in 1970 and 1973. His work confirms Autogenic Therapy as an extremely effective form of psychotherapy. The emphasis remains on allowing the self-righting mechanisms of mind and body, this time by using an extended exercise, and staying in it for as long as is necessary in a given session.

The term 'Autogenic Neutralisation' means the process by which the 'disturbing potency of neuronal record' can be released or discharged (neutralised). Luthe realised that the autogenic process somehow involved many different parts of the brain, in many cases allowing the subject to revisit past traumas and re-encounter the senses and feelings involved. It is clear that, given the right opportunity, the brain knows exactly what it needs to do to achieve true healing.

Luthe began to use one of the early autogenic exercises with his patients — this time in a different setting. The work is done individually, the subject lying on a couch, covered with a blanket, and the room is darkened. This reduces stimuli linked with surroundings, and allows the autogenic state to be prolonged. After completion of the exercise, the subject would stay in the autogenic state, and be encouraged to adopt an attitude of '*carte blanche*'. This state allowed the mind and body to open up to any feelings or physical sensations which might be around. Sometimes it is hard for the subject to let go of preconceived ideas, so at first they may try to direct the brain consciously.

Case 1 — Mary

Mary was 36, with a young family. After learning basic AT, she was left with disturbing issues of anger and grief, which she wanted to explore further. She describes her first neutralisation session: 'When the exercise finished, I lay there wondering quite what I was doing. Nothing seemed to be happening. Where were all the dramatic pictures about my family/parents — all the things I'm "supposed to be confronting"? The therapist would gently ask me what was happening, and I would reply, "Nothing". After I suppose about twenty minutes, I said, dismissively and irritated: "All I can see is one of my piano pupils — struggling with his scales." My therapist said, "Tell me about him." I began to describe him — how sad it was that he had such difficulty flowing with music; how he couldn't express himself, and playing the piano was for him not a channel through which to find himself. I began to cry, as I realised that I was describing some aspects of myself. The session quickly moved on — plenty of images of family, etc., and, months later, I realised that my brain had done exactly as Luthe described it would in a first session. It had given me access to myself (all unsuspecting through an unrelated person), and then gone on to give an overview of much of the work my brain needed to do over several months. But I had tried to ignore this at first — trying to "edit" my session with ill-placed judgement.'

As it became clear that it was necessary for the subject to speak, in order to describe sensations and scenarios as they occurred, and to 'move things on', Luthe began to tape-record the sessions, and this became an important therapeutic tool. The subject was encouraged to bring their own cassette-tape, and take it home to transcribe and analyse for themselves.

It was clear that the timing of the session was self-governing, and this was respected. Luthe found that the period of time that a subject needed to engage in the process varied. The session could take as little as fifteen minutes or as long as two hours, the ending usually following a neutral period of inactivity, then a positive feeling that 'all is right with the world'. The therapist needed to be aware of the possible session structure, recognising the timing of its conclusion, in order to avoid inappropriate interruption and possible distress for the subject afterwards.

Generally there is little quiet dialogue during the session. The therapist remains very much outside the process — merely acting as witness to it, and, in the early sessions, acknowledging the subject's progress while they are establishing themselves in using the technique. The therapist's only intervention is a technical one — managing the tape-recorder, establishing that the subject is comfortable, facilitating the process. Above all, the therapist does not interfere or direct proceedings, but instead develops a sense of timing and appropriateness in this work, which experience is then passed on to the subject, who is able to continue by themselves at home. So, sessions which may have begun on a weekly or fortnightly basis with the therapist might continue monthly or, perhaps, bi-monthly, with the subject working on their own in between.

When therapeutic work is as unstructured as autogenic neutralisation inevitably is, it is easy to expect that it will all be focused on past trauma. Certainly working through this material is how resolution comes about, but the process is often far from negative. Often people revisit 'good times' which had been 'forgotten'. Memories of old friends, scenarios of childhood treats, etc., can all play their part in a neutralisation session, just as they can in basic AT.

RESISTANCE

Sometimes the subject is clearly resisting their own processes, and the therapist needs to recognise whether the resistance is 'brain-facilitating' or 'brain-antagonising', in order to help them overcome this. Often the therapist merely offers reassurance, simply by stating that all is well in the room, and they are there to help.

Brain-Facilitating Resistance

This type of resistance actively helps the brain in its processes. To engage in the topic by forcing it could lead to distress if resolution cannot be achieved. This is generally understood to be a positive form of resistance — where interference in the process, or avoidance of engaging in aspects of it during a session, is the right course. The therapist's skill allows for this — respecting that when this type of resistance shows up, it is all right to leave the topic alone. Themes emerge which can grow from a brief mention in one session to further elaboration in subsequent sessions. There is a mutual trust that when the time is right — perhaps when the subject is feeling stronger, and the topic returns — it can be broached.

Brain-Antagonising Resistance

Trusting in the brain's self-righting mechanisms is always the key in all autogenic work. If the subject consciously steers away from a topic, they are resisting the brain's natural moves towards resolution. For example, in a neutralising session, there may be strong feelings around, and it might feel too uncomfortable to continue. The subject may sit up and open their eyes suddenly, in distress, in the middle of off-loading. In this situation, they are interrupting the process, which, if left unresolved, could leave them distressed and suffering from unpleasant psychosomatic symptoms. They have consciously avoided the issue, antagonising the brain's natural impulse. The therapist's task is to help them regain trust in their own processes — reassuring them that all is well in the room, acknowledging the difficulty, and letting them know that it is all right to explore or 'go with' the issue and attendant feelings.

Guilt and Forgiveness
The power of allowing the self to work with the self is evident in the next story.

Case 2 — Zola

Zola was aged 58. With her family grown up, her marriage problems were thrown into stark reality. During one neutralisation session, she revisited all the occasions where she had done or thought 'wrong' as regards her marriage. There had been plenty of expressions of anger and frustration in previous sessions, but this time Zola seemed to be tearing herself apart with guilt. She had returned from a holiday with a girlfriend, and her session returned to that holiday and others from the past. She needed to express her guilt feelings, and she did, by crying and asking unanswerable questions of 'What if?' Near the end of the session, she became very quiet, then said: 'There's music. It's the last movement of the St John Passion by Bach.' The therapist asked what it was saying to her, and she didn't know. The therapist asked how she was feeling, and the reply was: 'It's lovely — it is very peaceful and serene.' She stayed with that feeling, and with the music, and the session ended. When she looked up the music later, it was a chorus with the words: 'Rest here in peace, Redeemer blest and holy, Henceforth no more will I bewail thee, and lead thou me to peace.' (Translations vary from original German.)

It is fair to say that neutralisation takes place from the very first moment that a person starts using basic AT. This is especially so in the case of post-traumatic stress disorder (PTSD). The following case vividly describes this, but the young man was not able to continue with AT at the time. Although he recognised that it was certainly going to do the job, he could not face doing it right then.

Case 3 — Anthony

Anthony was a young man who, as a car passenger, had survived a motorway pile-up where several people had died. Two years after the event, Anthony was left with severe anxiety, which prevented him from functioning in any kind of normal way. He could remember nothing at all of the accident, and knew that he would have to if he was to rid himself of his symptoms. Other treatment had so far been unsuccessful and he came to learn AT. After the first session, when he had just been using short-stitch, he told the following story: 'I had a dream — it was of the car crashing. I was strapped in my seat and I couldn't move. The car was veering everywhere, crashing into other cars on the icy road. I thought each time it crashed that I would be dead. I heard the screams of a woman passenger. I must have lost consciousness. I woke up from the dream in a cold sweat. Next day, I was very upset, and couldn't stop telling people what had happened. I know it was a good thing, but I was very scared by it.' Anthony's autogenic therapist asked him what had happened after the dream — did he get up and drink a bottle of brandy? Did he wake up someone else? Did he distract himself? 'I turned over and went back to sleep,' he replied. His therapist was astonished.

This demonstrates the brain's need to unload specific details, to release the memory in order to neutralise the disturbing feelings. Here was an extraordinary example of the self-normalising properties of the autogenic method. Despite the trauma of revisiting the accident in a dream, Anthony was able to go to sleep again.

CREATIVITY MOBILISATION TECHNIQUE (CMT)

A further development of Dr Luthe's, from the 1940s, CMT uses painting as the medium of expression. The method involves doing

'Mess Painting' several times a week for about two months. It can follow a basic AT course but it can also stand alone. It serves 'well people who want to be weller' (Virginia Goldstein, *The Magic of Mess Painting,* 1999).

THE PURPOSE OF CMT

The method helps people to get in touch with feelings and memories, through letting go of convention or effort. Using primary colours creates an avenue of emotional access which allows movement of feeling. It can help to boost all artistic endeavours, whatever medium: painting, writing, music, dance, drama, pottery, sculpture, etc. It can also help to alleviate psychosomatic symptoms.

The challenges of this course are considerable, involving not only the painting sessions, but also keeping a diary and checklist of feelings. After the session, the subject has a bath — a time for reflection on the day's process.

The CMT course is usually done in a group, but the painting is carried out alone, at home. The idea is to create deliberate mess, which has no form or intent, and is analysed only by the subject, not the therapist. At least fifteen paintings are done in each session, of which there are four per week. Then, a minimum of sixty paintings are taken to the weekly session. Each person will have prepared their 'showing', selecting particular paintings for presentation and explanation to the group and therapist.

THE PAINTING SESSION

- *The Tools.* These consist of powder paints of eight colours (red, blue, yellow, green, purple, brown, black and white) mixed with starch, a separate container and half-inch brush for each colour, and an unlimited supply of broad-sheet newspaper, numbered in advance. Also needed is a drying rack, so that each sheet can dry while the next paintings are done.
- *The Environment.* This is dedicated to the painting if possible. This may be in a garage or shed, or a spare room. Sometimes the difficulties in creating the right environment are very off-

putting, and yet it is surprising how committed people can be as they get to grips with yards of plastic sheeting stuck to walls for weeks on end. Indeed, for some it is necessary to keep dismantling the environment only to remake it for the next session.

The aim of the session, once begun, is to be as continuous and flowing as possible. Newspaper is used so that there are no inhibitions about fresh, virgin paper — it is easier to create 'mess' on paper that is going to be thrown out. The paper is big enough to allow big expansive gestures — full arm movements are encouraged. It is important that no 'margins' are observed — the brush strokes should spill over the edge of the paper. The intention is to make a series of 'no-thought' mess-paintings, covering 70–90 per cent of the newspaper in several colours.

Two minutes are spent on each painting, which is then moved straight on to a drying rack, and another sheet is started quickly. Brushes are chosen at random — no thought given to form, shape or colour. The paintings are done with no conscious concern for beauty or result. There should be plenty of physical movement, and variation in application is often evident — for example, throwing spots of colour; smearing with the fingers; tearing the paper (with anger?) During the session, any feelings that may emerge should be expressed — spontaneous singing, laughing, crying, shouting, swearing. The bath afterwards is a time to reflect, and the diary should be written after that.

As time goes on, the emergence of powerful and beautiful abstract paintings often surprises the participants. The paintings can be mounted on card and viewed behind glass for their full impact. Often people will hang them in their home for a certain period. This acknowledges their work, and the expression of themselves.

Virginia Goldstein (in California) is acknowledged as the world's expert in CMT. In the UK, Vera Diamond, who has studied CMT with Luthe, occasionally runs small group or individual courses.

CHAPTER 12

AUDIT AND RESEARCH

O ver the years, very many (reputedly over 3,000) scientific papers have been published, which document the effectiveness of Autogenic Therapy. Some of the methods used have been found to be non-standard (as far as the UK and Ireland go), but overall, the efficacy of AT has been proven in many areas. It is not in the remit of this book to list all available research literature — this can be found elsewhere.

Studies have been done in countries as diverse as Italy, Russia and Japan, as well as Schultz's and others' original work in Germany, and Luthe's in Canada. Unfortunately, only a limited amount is available in English. We will include here just a small sample of the more up-to-date studies.

AT AND ASTHMA

Environmental, physical and emotional stress may well be the main precipitating factors in asthma attacks.

M. Henry and others[1] conducted a study of two groups of asthmatic patients. Over an eight-month period, one group was treated with Autogenic Therapy, while the control group was treated with supportive group psychotherapy. The AT group showed significant clinical improvement in respiratory function. No significant improvement was noted in the control group.

CARDIO-PROTECTIVE EFFECTS OF AT

Dr Malcolm Carruthers MD, FRCPath did research in this area. Two controlled trials found significant reductions in a wide range of cardiovascular risk factors in response either to Autogenic Training or physical training. Results in the AT users showed:

- Reduction in the use of medication such as tranquillisers, sleeping pills and anti-hypertensives
- Lowering of cholesterol levels, tryglicerides and free fatty acids
- Reduction in pulse rate
- Reduction of both systolic and diastolic blood pressure

AT AND ANXIETY

M. Farné and A. Corallo[2] conducted a study in Italy of seventy-nine patients suffering from anxiety, and a variety of physical symptoms related to stress. The trial group learned AT alongside a control group, where no intervention was made. There was some improvement in both groups after the initial consultation. This improvement continued only in the trial group. The outcome showed significant decrease in emotional distress and physical symptoms.

AT IN AIDS AND HIV

Dr K. Kermani[3] carried out a study of fifty AIDS and HIV patients, which showed considerable improvement in their quality of life and the development of a positive attitude towards the future. Control of symptoms such as pain, night sweats, diarrhoea and raised temperature was noted. These improvements were maintained by most patients for significant periods after the course.

AUTOGENIC TRAINING IN RHEUMATOID ARTHRITIS

A pilot study was conducted by Dr K. Chakravarty and others[4] at the Department of Rheumatology, Stoke Mandeville Hospital, Bucks. Previous research suggests the possible relationship between rheumatoid arthritis and psychological and emotional disturbance. In this study, fifteen patients with rheumatoid arthritis were taught AT. Twelve others acted as a control group. Pre- and post-course measurements were taken of pain, early morning stiffness, joint count and grip strength, as well as haematological and serological tests. Significant improvement was noted in all areas tested.

AT IN PREGNANCY AND LABOUR

Professor Prill, Department of Obstetrics, University of Warzburg, conducted several studies using AT to help women in labour. One study[5] involved 1,000 women, and showed significant advantages, including a reduction in the length of labour and a less distressing birth experience.

AT IN THE WORKPLACE

In a paper delivered at the World Congress of Psychiatry (No. 11) in August 1999, Professor Yuji Sasaki from Komazawa University, Japan, described a study introducing AT to 23,710 workers in fifty companies, from 1994 to 1996. Beneficial effects were experienced in the mental and physical health of the workers. This showed in a reduction of medical expenses, work accidents and suicide rates. In one bus company where the drivers had learnt AT, accident rates had fallen by two-thirds over four years, rendering one of the three 'accident managers' redundant.

AT AND MIGRAINE

The Letchworth Centre for Healthy Living conducted a trial for the Hertfordshire Health Agency with the support of a consultant neurologist at the Lister Hospital. Patients were referred by local GPs, and they were considered suitable for the study if they:

- had not responded well to drug treatment;
- experienced side effects that precluded the continued use of medication;
- preferred not to use regular medication;
- were self-motivated and compliant with the requirements of the course.

Christine Pinch taught AT to twenty-nine migraine sufferers. Twenty-one attended their follow-ups eight weeks after the end of the course, and completed a questionnaire.

The questionnaires showed that, in a significant majority, the frequency and severity of migraine was less, along with the need for analgesia; in many, the pattern of attacks had changed (indicating that the process was still ongoing); general health improved (sleep, coping better); visits to GP less often.

AUDIT OF AT COURSES

Dr Anne Bowden MB ChB, DHC, MFHom, DipAT created an audit of AT courses at the Royal London Homeopathic Hospital.

In 1992, 188 questionnaires were sent to all past AT trainees at the RLHH — 132 were returned. Most of the patients had physical or mental problems, which had not responded to conventional treatments.

The problems ranged from emotional (insomnia, stress/tension/anxiety, panic, depression) to physical (hypertension, headaches, pain, asthma, arthritis, eczema). Without including all the detail here, the general trend was towards significant improvement in all symptoms.

Additional improvements included:

- Feeling more positive/in control/assertive
- Feeling able to relax
- Coping better
- Feeling emotionally stronger
- Being able to communicate/'speak my mind'
- Living in the present (not dreading the future)
- Feeling accepting of self (no longer self-blaming)
- Feeling less irritable.

According to Dr Bowden: *'Probably the most important result was a sense of regaining control of themselves through relaxation, and the development of new confidence and a sense of well-being.'*

REFERENCES

(1) Henry M., J.L.G. De Rivera, I.J. Gonzalez-Martin, and J. Abreu (1993), 'Improvement of Respiratory Function in Chronic Asthmatic Patients with Autogenic Therapy' *Journal of Psychosomatic Research*, Vol. 37, no. 3, pp. 265–70.

(2) Farné M. and A. Corallo (1992), 'Autogenic Training and Signs of Distress: An Experimental Study', *Boll. Soc. It. Biol. Sper.*, N6-Vol. LXV111-Idelson-Napoli.

(3) Kermani Dr K. (1987), 'Stress, Emotions, Autogenic Training and AIDS: A Holistic Approach to the Management of HIV-infected Individuals', *Holistic Medicine*, Vol. 2, pp. 203–15.

(4) Chakravarty K., K. Murray and M. Webley (1992), 'Autogenic Training in Rheumatoid Arthritis — A Pilot Study', *British Journal of Rheumatology*, Abstr. Suppl. 31:1.

(5) Prill H.J. (1965), 'Das Autogenic Training in der Geburtshilfe and Gynakologie'

BIBLIOGRAPHY

Schultz J.L., W. Luthe, *Autogenic Therapy,* Vols 1–4. Grune & Stratton 1969 and 1970; British Autogenic Society 2001.

Luthe W., *Autogenic Therapy,* Vols 5 & 6. Grune & Stratton 1973; British Autogenic Society 2001.

O'Donovan, J.B., *Autogenic Training in Organic Illness – a handbook for therapists.* J.B. O'Donovan 1989.

Luthe W., *Workshop notes for Autogenic Training Therapist Course, Vol 1 1978, Vol 2 1982.*

RESOURCES

British Autogenic Society
Royal London Homœopathic Hospital
Great Ormond Street
London
WC1N 3HR

From June 2002 to Autumn 2004, while the Great Ormond Street site is being rebuilt, the temporary address is:

British Autogenic Society
Royal London Homœopathic Hospital
Greenwell Street
London
W1W 5BP

Email: autosoc@lineone.net

For a list of therapists, please send a stamped addressed envelope to the above address.

Or visit the website: autogenic-therapy.org.uk

In English-speaking countries where local organisations for Autogenic Therapy are not yet known, please contact the BAS as above. The Society's aim is to spread the availability of AT, and they can provide professional therapist training courses where enough health professionals are interested in a certain locality.

INDEX

Index